MANUFACTURED BODIES

The Impact of Industrialisation on London Health

Gaynor Western and Jelena Bekvalac

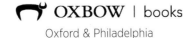

OXBOW | books

Oxford & Philadelphia

Published in the United Kingdom in 2020 by
OXBOW BOOKS
The Old Music Hall, 106–108 Cowley Road, Oxford, OX4 1JE

and in the United States by
OXBOW BOOKS
1950 Lawrence Road, Havertown, PA 19083

Paperback Edition: ISBN 978-1-78925-322-1
Digital Edition: ISBN 978-1-78925-323-8 (epub)

A CIP record for this book is available from the British Library

Library of Congress Control Number: 2019953216

Printed in the United Kingdom by Short Run Press, Exeter
Typeset by Frabjous Books

For a complete list of Oxbow titles, please contact:

United Kingdom
Oxbow Books
Telephone (01865) 241249
Email: oxbow@oxbowbooks.com
www.oxbowbooks.com

United States of America
Oxbow Books
Telephone (610) 853-9131, Fax (610) 853-9146
Email: queries@casemateacademic.com
www.casemateacademic.com/oxbow

Oxbow Books is part of the Casemate Group

Research project funded by the City of London Archaeological Trust (CoLAT) Rosemary Green Grant

Front Cover: Sculpture Anguish #6 by Seo Young Deok
Back cover: (left) Osteologist anatomically laying out skeletal remains © Museum of London
(right) Postcard of Fleet Street, London, Ludgate Hill and Circus, 19th century, © Museum of London

Dedicated to the memory of Bill White

Emeritus Curator, Centre for Human Bioarchaeology,
Museum of London

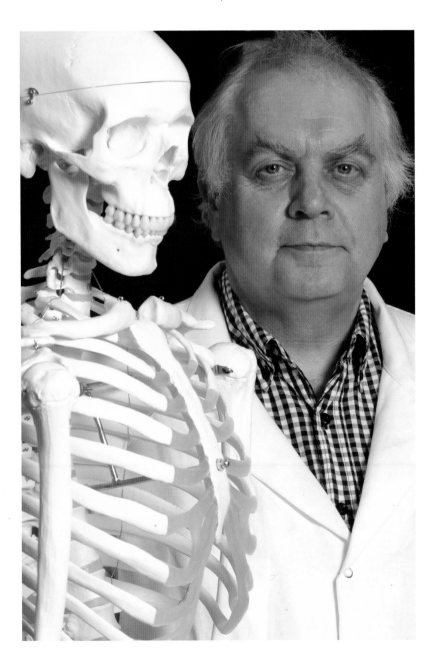

Contents

Acknowledgements

The research project and book would not have been possible without the generous funding from the Rosemary Green grant awarded by the City of London Archaeological Trust and we are most grateful to have been the recipients. We would like to thank the Museum of London; Museum of London Archaeology; Ossafreelance; Oxford Archaeology; Allen Archaeology; Wessex Archaeology; Worcestershire Archaeology; AOC Archaeology; University of Bradford; University of Durham and York Archaeology; English Heritage (Dr Simon Mays); Historic England (Kevin Booth) and the Reverend Canon Dr Alison Joyce and church team at St Bride's Church, Fleet Street who all helped enable the research to come to fruition with enabling access to skeletal collections and to Anthea Boylston, Dr Simon Mays, Dr Anwen Cafell, Dr Louise Loe, Stephen Rowland, Dr Andy Boucher (Headland Archaeology) and James Langthorne (Pre Construct Archaeology) for generously sharing osteological data. We thank Professor Margaret Cox and Professor Charlotte Roberts for kindly allowing us to access and use the Bills of Mortality data from their publication. The digital radiography

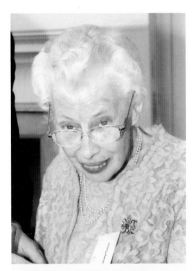

Photograph of Rosemary Green
Supplied by the City of London Archaeological Trust.

was made possible through Reveal Imaging Ltd and we thank them for carrying out the digital radiography and to Dr Ross Kendall, Ergian Musto, Anna Skaar and the masters' students provided by Malin Holst from University of York who kindly assisted at various locations throughout the project with the preparation of the skeletal elements to be radiographed. Our thanks to David Allan for working his way through the many radiographs generated, sharing his radiological expertise, and his valuable analytical input. We were fortunate to be able to carry out CT scanning and thank Dr Indran Davagnanam, London Neuroimaging Specialists Ltd for making that possible and to Dr Natasha Davendralingam for her work in rendering and remodelling the scans. Thanks to photographers Richard Stroud and John Chase, Museum of London for adding to the rich collection of images in the book, Richard Dabb in the Picture Library and Dr Rebecca Redfern Museum of London, for her encouragement. Special thanks to Dr Rebecca Gowland for giving her time to read the first draft and her comments. Last and by no means least our heartfelt thanks to our families who have supported us throughout, Annette Bekvalac, Patricia Fox and particularly Patricia Western who have been subjected to the glories of all of the chapters.

Foreword

One day in 2004 or 2005, I was at my desk in the Museum of London when the telephone rang. It was a lady who identified herself as Rosemary Green, a retired librarian then living in Poole, Dorset. Was I the secretary of the City of London Archaeological Trust? Yes I was. Did the Trust take bequests? I sat up. Yes we did. And so our association with Rosemary Green began.

When she died in 2012, Rosemary Green made substantial bequests to five charities: the City of London Archaeological Trust (CoLAT), the Friends of City Churches, the Historic Churches Trust, the Postal Heritage Trust and the Philatelic Society. These charities evidently represented some of her main interests.

CoLAT, founded by the Museum of London and the Corporation of London in 1974, is a charity whose purpose is to obtain funds for and to encourage all kinds of archaeological work in the City of London and its environs. Since the expansion in provision for archaeological excavation and research by developers since the 1980s, reinforced by legislation since 1990, CoLAT has directed its modest funding towards support for non-professional groups and for academic research in all periods of London's archaeology and history when connected to archaeological discoveries. In the case of the Rosemary Green bequest, the Trust decided to fund one outstanding piece of research, a project lasting up to three years, and invited applications. There were several of note; and the award went to *The Impact of Industrialisation on London Health*, a collaborative research project with Jelena Bekvalac at the Centre for Human Bioarchaeology, Museum of London and Gaynor Western, Ossafreelance.

This is what they said they would do:

> a new research project based upon the analysis of the archaeological human skeletal remains of 2,500 individuals hopes to uncover new clues about how the nature of disease affecting the UK's population has changed over the past millennium. Modern health trends have seen a shift towards increasing life expectancy but also what are often thought of as 'man-made' conditions such

as obesity and cancer. Given our technologically driven lifestyles today, far removed from the more physically active, organic existence of the majority of our forebears, there are questions about the origins of these diseases and how they relate to the modern environment. Are these diseases genuinely recent or is it that they couldn't be identified before? To what extent is our modern, artificial environment responsible for the diseases that we experience today? How has the industrialisation of modern society impacted on our health?

Let me add two notes about the way we view the context. The historian Eric Hobsbawm has written that 'The Industrial Revolution marks the most fundamental transformation of human life in the history of the world recorded in written documents'.[1] Archaeologists and their colleagues who specialise in the study of human skeletons have, especially since the 1980s, excavated and studied thousands of skeletons from churchyards, crypts and half-forgotten cemetery sites beneath modern buildings. Health and disease in the Industrial period is now becoming understood, all over Britain.[2]

This is the starting-point for the study, funded by the bequest of Rosemary Green, which follows.

John Schofield
Secretary, City of London Archaeological Trust
2019

[1] E. Hobsbawm, *Industry and Empire* (1990), 14.
[2] C. Roberts and M. Cox, *Health and Disease in Britain: From Prehistory to the Present Day* (2003), 287–358.

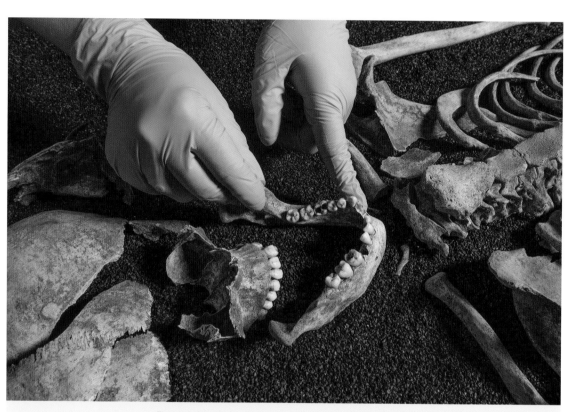

Figure 1 Osteologist anatomically laying out skeletal remains

(© Museum of London)

Introduction

When every part of the machine is correctly adjusted and in perfect harmony, health will hold dominion over the human organism.

A. T. Still, MD, DO (1828–1917)

We read about it and hear about it on TV every day. We're getting fatter. We're consuming too much sugar. Cancer rates are soaring. We are less active in our sedentary jobs but the roads are busier, with fatal accidents occurring on a daily basis. The climate is changing and air pollution is getting worse. These blights of modern lifestyles in the UK are a constant source of discussion and concern, the almost inescapable consequences of our revolutionised way of living surrounded by machines, technology and convenience foods. On the other hand, medicine is advancing, we are successfully treating more conditions than ever and we are living longer, though that's not without its problems. The impact of industrialisation and how this has shaped health and healthcare today is, then, a fundamental consideration for understanding the role of our living environments in causing disease. Is industrialisation and the connected technology-dependent modernisation of our occupations, diets and lifestyles really the cause of the health issues we see today? When did these diseases first occur? Were they absent in the past or is it the case that we just aren't aware of any evidence for them?

At the centre of the modern day fast-paced drive for speed, wealth and medical innovations in the UK is London. By the 1700s, London was not only the largest city in Europe but also half of England's urban population lived there. E. A. Wrigley once said that London life was 'qualitatively and quantitatively different from the rest of England', 'a force promoting the modernisation of English society'. Its unique place in history within the wider setting of Great Britain as a hub for exchange, of not only traded goods but of people and knowledge, has propelled the generation of a living environment with individual demands and consequences for its inhabitants' health. This is most abundantly clear in the pivotal era of London's rapid expansion that sparked our modern way of living: the Industrial Period. This era, spanning between *c.* 1750 and 1900, was dominated by the aim of improving manufacturing efficiency in order to generate increasing amounts of wealth. In turn, industrialisation led to society becoming more and more dependent upon technology to generate the necessary foods and materials required to keep up with the needs of the exponentially growing population. Technological innovations were often highly experimental during this period, with little known of their long term consequences. Not only that, manual labour was still a huge part of the process of industrialisation, with many jobs only partly aided by mechanical equipment. The scale of industrialisation was vast, requiring a whole new network of infrastructure to move food and goods in and out of London, either to the rest of the UK or overseas, by road, rail track, canals, rivers or by sea. These unprecedented engineering and manufacturing feats were physically demanding tasks requiring hundreds of thousands of labourers in the City and beyond.

At the same time, the rural economy was changing with similar aspirations of producing more wealth. Many tenant farmers faced eviction and migration to the cities to earn wages, rather than being able to continue to produce their own means of subsistence. In London, the material divides between the 'haves' and 'have-nots' became more and more stark. Many of the labouring classes were forced to endure cramped and poor quality housing in the City, while working extremely long hours in ill-ventilated workshops, warehouses and factories. Without the legal protections or safety regulations that we take for granted today, pollution and workplace hazards went unchecked and many people found themselves working in desperate conditions. In comparison, wealthier areas such as Chelsea and Hackney progressed with their superior houses, their occupants engaged in fine dining and occasionally strolling into town or about pleasure gardens for shopping, pastries and tea. These social divisions had serious and shocking consequences on health and life expectancy. Chadwick's survey of 1842 concluded that life expectancy for labourers and servants in London was just 22 years compared to 45 years for the gentry and professional classes.

While the living and working environments deteriorated for many in London, medical understanding and treatment was advancing. During the Industrial period, 'occupational' diseases were first recognised and studied, and for the first time micro-organisms were observed and identified as the cause of infectious diseases. In fact, the severity of the conditions brought about by the Industrial Revolution led to the instigation of some of the first 'medical epidemiology' studies, where local environments and the pathogens contained within them were mapped to identify regional differences in outbreaks of infectious disease. The understanding of the combined role that poor ventilation, over-crowded conditions, polluted air and pathogens contributed to disease had a significant impact on the way disease processes were understood and remedied. By improving living standards in combination with developing vaccinations, many common killers of the Industrial period were all but annihilated to the point where it is now considered by epidemiologists that we entered a new age of pathology at the turn of the 20th century, transitioning from infectious to non-communicable diseases as the major causes of ill-health and death. The end of the Industrial Period therefore marked the end of an era in human pathology.

Although the control that we now have over many previously fatal infectious diseases is plain to us today, studying disease in the past can be problematic. Medical terminology and understanding have changed rapidly and continue to do so. Historical records are a relatively recent phenomenon and even those that we do have are often incomplete or have been inconsistently maintained by people with different understandings and using different words to describe diseases and causes of death. Diagnosis based on the inadequate methods of medical observation at the time was at best, imprecise. Surgery and the observation of the internal body parts of patients was extremely limited until the very late 19th and early 20th centuries following the invention of general anaesthesia, although human anatomical and pathological dissection of the deceased had provided a limited source of knowledge for medical studies from the Tudor period onwards.

Medical imaging, at the time known as 'skiagraphy' or the 'drawing of shadows', only took its first steps towards being the vital diagnostic tool it is today in London in 1896, a year after the discovery of x-rays in Bavaria by Wilhelm Röntgen. Without a solid source of direct evidence from the past, therefore, it is very difficult to objectively assess historical frequencies of diseases.

In recent years, the development of commercial archaeology has led to a series of excavations of cemeteries and burial grounds dating to the Industrial period throughout the UK, in advance of development of sites by building contractors. The archaeological recording of human skeletal remains by professionally trained osteoarchaeologists and their subsequent retention in museum archives provides a unique opportunity to understand crucial aspects of health in the past that help crystallize our understanding of health in the present. This in turn informs us about the potential for future health outcomes. Large samples of human skeletal remains available for scientific study can hold the key to our understanding of disease in the past because they form a body of hard evidence that can be examined using newly developing techniques, both now and in the future. This is particularly relevant in our attempts to further our understanding of the role of living and working environments in health outcomes according to geographic locations and their specific local settings. By comparing and contrasting the health of Londoners over time to inhabitants of other areas in the UK, we get a very real sense of how living in the environment of the largest metropolis in Great Britain affected lives in the past and continues to do so today.

The opportunity provided by the Rosemary Green grant, awarded by the City of London Archaeological Trust (CoLAT) in 2015, has allowed osteoarchaeologists at the Museum of London for the first time to analyse the skeletal remains of almost 2300 individuals from numerous sites across Britain using digital radiography and CT (computerised tomography) scans, providing more detailed images. We have therefore been able to explore current themes in health today using modern clinical diagnostic methods to examine the independent skeletal evidence, asking questions of the digital data concerning the big news topics of today, such as accidents and trauma, air pollution, cancer, obesity and ageing. Industrialisation was not a uniform process and had different impacts according to local environments, natural resources and the demands of implementing new nationwide infrastructure. The aim of the research was therefore to look at the health of Londoners over time and to see how this compared to more rurally located towns and villages, putting London in its wider context. By using this new digital image archive in combination with existing osteological records, we have been able to investigate some previously unsolved questions, giving us a new and fascinating insight into the history of the health of Londoners up to the present day.

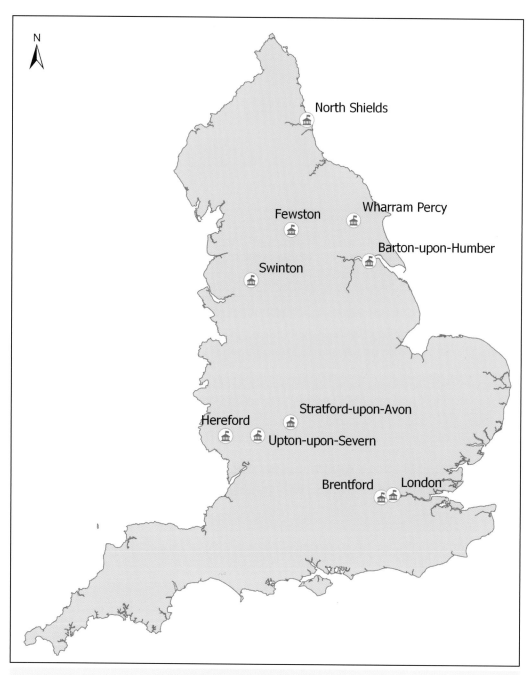

Figure 2 National sites in relation to London

Gazetteer of sites

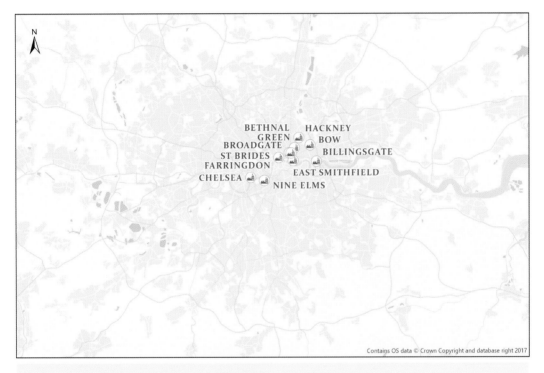

Figure 3 Sites in London

London industrial sites (*c.* 1750–1900)

Bethnal Green and Spitalfields Bethnal Green was an East End hamlet of Stepney, neighbouring the parish of Spitalfields, until 1743, when it was made into a separate parish. Consisting of 755 acres (305.5 ha), due to its vast expansion the parish subsequently became a metropolitan borough in 1900 and then part of the London Borough of Tower Hamlets in 1965. The earliest recorded settlement dates to the 12th and 13th centuries when 'the Green' consisted of a village common and a cluster of tenanted wooden framed cottages, located on former marshland and forest. Nearby was the Bishop's Hall, a hunting lodge. Bethnal Green was part of the highway from Mile End to Cambridge Heath and Hackney in the 1580s and, as such, was an important passing point for large numbers of cattle and heavy carriages. The open area of the Green outside of the City was used by wealthy London merchants as a country retreat. From about 1650, businessmen then began to buy up copyhold leases and to rent lands out or develop them for housing. Many of the new houses were very small, only 13–19 ft (c. 4–5.8 m) across, designed to be let out to the weavers who were spilling out of Spitalfields into Bethnal Green as the Huguenot textile industry boomed. Spitalfields had a long history with cloth production and some of the open land about here owned by the priory was known as the 'Tesell' or teasel ground, planted to be used by textile workers to rough up the nap on cloth. Already by 1711, Bethnal Green was populated by around 8496 people, rapidly growing to 10,877 people by 1831, by which time there was little open area between the individual hamlets. The population density and its increasing poverty made the area unpopular with wealthier Londoners (Fig. 4). By now, Bethnal Green had become synonymous with the 'labouring poor' and regular typhus outbreaks caused by stagnant water, rubbish, animals in backyards, dust-heaps, and leaking cess pits. One particular

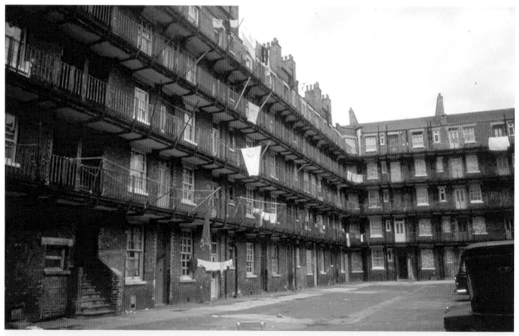

Figure 4 Lolesworth Buildings, Thrawl Street built by the East End Dwellings Co Ltd. in 1885
(cc-by-sa/2.0 - © Derek Voller geograph.org.uk/p/1755278)

hotspot for grime and crime in Bethnal Green was an area of narrow alleyways and over-run housing known as The Nichol, where the death rate in 1886–1888 was 40 in 1000 compared to 22.8 for Bethnal Green overall and 18.4 for the whole of London.

Local trades included brick makers, tailors, costermongers, shoe makers, dustmen, sawyers, carpenters and cabinet makers, rope makers, brewers and silk weavers, though some 'traditional' trades were covers for thieves and prostitutes. Ship repair was also a major industry. Several factories existed by 1838, especially serving the furniture and cloth industries, and continued to expand until the 1930s and '40s. Local markets continued to thrive and expand, however, until the recent redevelopment of Spitalfields, which to this point has retained many of its large historic buildings, attracting artists and musicians as residents. In contrast, slum clearance of Bethnal Green began in the 1920s by the London County Council (LCC), who in addition to The Bethnal Green and East London Housing Association, attempted to provide new, clean, affordable housing. The combination of slum clearance, the separation of residential from occupational areas and intensive bombing during the Second World War forced the relocation of most factories out of the area. By the 1950s, private leasing, a lack of council housing provision and dispersal of the old community caused by the rehousing of 40,000 people by the LCC led to a second wave of criminality, resulting in the Vallance Road headquarters being set up by the notorious Kray brothers. The East End docks closed in the 1980s and the area has undergone a series of regeneration projects aimed at tackling the continuing poverty in the area.

Bow was also known as 'Stratford-le-Bow' because it was the location of a rare bridge, arched like a bow, connecting Bow to Stratford. Originally surrounded by marshland and consisting of about 465 acres (188 ha) of land, the area supported arable and pasture subsistence as well as nursery gardens, some of which grew exotic plants (Figure 5). At this time, Bow was described as a rural idyll with its 'cornfields, pastures and pleasant meadows' by Samuel Pepys. Like Bethnal Green, the hamlet of Bow was separated from Stepney in about 1720. In its earlier history, Bow was a centre for calico printing and bakery as well as scarlet dying for the *East India Company* but these trades had largely died out by 1795.

A substantial pottery factory was founded, producing Bow porcelain via a newly devised method of manufacture developed by Thomas Frye (1710–1762). At its peak, the factory owned by Messrs Crowther and Weatherby, where Frye was the works manager, employed 300 people including 90 painters. The factory only survived for about 20 years, however, after which other smaller businesses such as locksmiths, safe makers, paint, colour and varnish manufacturers continued to provide local trade

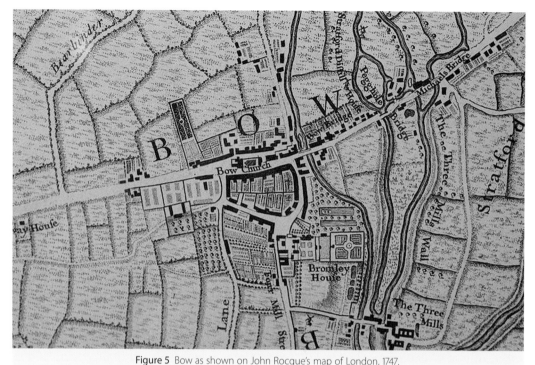

Figure 5 Bow as shown on John Rocque's map of London, 1747.

in addition to markets such as the Goose Fair, which was banned in the mid-19th century due to its rowdiness. One of the best known factories in the area was *Bryant and May* founded in 1861 after their partnership was formed in 1850 in Tooley Street, in Southwark (south of the River Thames), to import Swedish matches. The strike by the London Matchgirls at the factory in 1888, for better working conditions and concern over the associated condition 'Phossy Jaw', caused by the white phosphorous used on the matches is well documented. Eventually, white phosphorous was banned by the international *Berne Convention* in 1906 but the movement for women's rights led by Sylvia Pankhurst and the Suffragettes continued with Bow as a focus for a further 12 years. Bow continued very much in the same vein as Bethnal Green, being run by the Krays in the 1950s and '60s. More recently, extensive urban regeneration was undertaken at Bow following the Olympic Games that were held at neighbouring Stratford, which has provided new affordable homes fuelled by green technologies.

Chelsea is a location that has long been associated with wealth, though its early origins were comparably modest and rustic as part of a manor replete with meadow and pasture for cattle, sheep and pigs, and fields of barley, oats wheat and rye. Enclosure of the fields saw reduction of the common land, the last of which was removed in about 1810. In the 16th and 17th centuries the land was leased out in plots and was home to the states of Henry VIII, Thomas More and other courtiers who needed to find residences outside of nearby but overcrowded Westminster and Whitehall. During this time, an increasing amount of the land was used for market gardening and orchards to supply the demand in London for more locally grown fruit and vegetables. In 1605, The *Gardeners' Company of London* was founded to regulate the surging new trade. The area continued to attract wealthy merchants and gentlemen, leading to the construction of fine mansions. Chelsea was not without social problems. Many local tradesmen and working class residents lived in old, run down cottages and hovels in narrow streets and mews areas. Crime was a frequently reported problem. Nonetheless, Chelsea became a riverside resort for the wealthy and, later on, for the artistic. The gravels in the river bank created an easy landing spot and thus Chelsea became not only a convenient site for connecting to other parishes along the river, but also an important ferry crossing point.

The growing number of affluent building projects during the 19th century came at the cost of local market gardening trade, with the land being turned over for construction (Fig. 6). Nursery gardens furnishing the gentry with exotic plants and trees did survive but even this succumbed to housing expansion in the early 20th century. Wharves had been established by the 14th century and the ability to trade by river promoted local industries, such as glass making, silk production, porcelain, metalwork, paper-staining and brewing. More service industries started to develop during the 19th century, including the famous innovative plumbing and sanitation solutions of *Thomas Crapper and Company*, although they subsequently relocated to Stratford-upon-Avon. However, with the increasing number of well-off residents along the now aspirational King's Road came the growth of local retailing and professional occupations during the late 19th and 20th centuries, becoming the centre for fashion boutiques in the 'Swinging Sixties'.

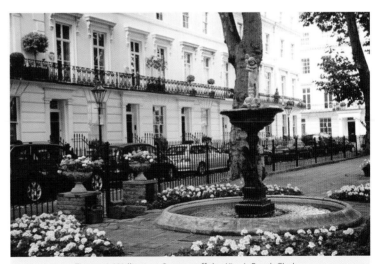

Figure 6 Wellington Square, off the King's Road, Chelsea
(cc-by-sa/2.0 - © D Williams – geograph.org.uk/p/3722)

Hackney Mare Street in Hackney was a distinct settlement by 1593, located along the route to Bethnal Green via Cambridge Heath, which was common pastureland. The hamlet consisted of timber-framed buildings including a staging post at the *Flying Horse Inn* but was still a small and remote settlement, with only 23 residents in 1605. Nonetheless, the area attracted wealthy, high status residents living in large houses situated in open pasturelands, including that of the City chamberlain Sir Thomas Player, which had 14 hearths. Despite its originally modest size, by 1720, Mare Street was the most populous district in the parish and houses lined both sides of the street, though they were still set in their own individual plots of land. By 1780, development on the east side of Mare Street set in motion a series of further house building that eventually ran continuously from Cambridge Heath to Hackney. Residents were very wealthy, including clergymen, academics and businessmen (Fig. 7).

By 1827, the road layout had to be improved to allow traffic to flow more freely and house building continued apace until 1860, when development had filled all the open spaces except for the garden of St Thomas' Square and the disused graveyards at St Thomas' place and the Congregational Chapel. The introduction of the new railway

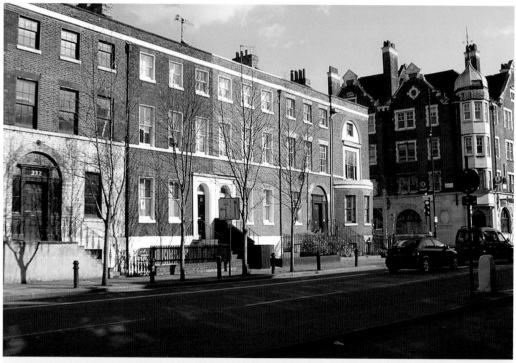

Figure 7 Mare Street, Hackney.
(Credit: Kockafej, GFDL-cc-by-sa/3.0 https://hu.wikipedia.org/wiki/F%C3%A1jl:Hackney_Mare_Street.jpg)

led to further construction in 1872. Socially, the area still had 'well-to-do' residents but several neighbouring streets were very poor. The prosperity of the area continued to decline. Factories were built from around 1903 when the area's popularity as an affluent residential area waned. Slum clearance was undertaken in the 1930s around the London Fields area followed by further compulsory purchases around Thomas Square, leading to its demolition. Large complexes and multi-storeyed building projects commenced. Today, most of Mare Street consists of 'non-descript low rise factories, shops and institutional buildings' and only a small strip of the original buildings from 12–20 Mare Street survive.

Nine Elms, situated in the Battersea, Vauxhall and Wandsworth areas of London, was traditionally a market gardening area consisting of about 300 acres (*c.* 120 ha) of land, supporting a number of horticulturalists and migrant labourers, especially females, travelling in from as far afield as Shropshire and north Wales (Fig. 8). In the late medieval period, horticulture in London became a profitable occupation and stemmed the need to import fruit and vegetables from neighbouring Holland. A fort was constructed here during the English Civil War (1642–3). Only after the building of a bridge at Battersea across the Thames did the parish of Nine Elms begin to expand with new houses but, due to the richness of the soils and pasture, construction development was slow and Battersea Fields was still a well-known open area in 1830.

Later in 1855, 320 acres (*c.* 130 ha) of fields purchased by the Commissioners of Works finally opened as a landscaped park, known as Vauxhall Pleasure Gardens, complete with cricket and tennis facilities, wooded walks and drives, a tropical garden, a gymnasium and an artificial lake, all thronged by crowds entertained by a

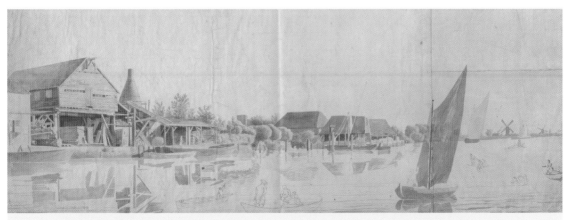

Figure 8 A wood yard on the Thames at Nine Elms, undated watercolour sketch by Samuel Scott (1702–1772).
(Credit: Yale Center for British Art https://collections.britishart.yale.edu/vufind/Record/1670326)

whole host of circus acts. The area was first served by an intercity train line running to Southampton in 1838, with local transport into the City consisting of coaches, omnibuses and trams. From the mid-19th century the area became urbanised and rapidly expanded according to this improved connectivity. In 1865, gasworks were built but subsequently devastated by the largest explosion in 19th century London. A million cubic feet of gas was ignited, killing 11 men. The railway was closed in 1948, having been damaged by the Blitz during the Second World War, but was replaced by New Covent Garden's flower and fruit and vegetable market in 1974, supplying 40% of the fresh fruit and vegetables to local vendors in London.

St Bride's, Farringdon Without is the historic centre of London, including Middle and Inner Temple, Chancery Lane, Smithfield and St. Bart's Hospital. The area became synonymous with the gold trade in the medieval period but the presence of the Fleet Ditch also attracted more low status industries such as tanners and curriers. The Ditch was little more than an open sewer and the land in its immediate vicinity was home to slums. Eventually, the river was culverted and Farringdon Street was constructed over it. Here, the busy Fleet Market subsequently opened in 1737 and sold meat, fish and vegetables. During the 18th and 19th centuries, Farringdon without was a densely packed mix of medieval and more modern buildings with substantial Victorian infrastructure superimposed on the preceding town layout. Much of the housing was constructed for the middle classes and consisted of large impressive town houses but

small courts and alleyways off the main streets also provided cheaper dwellings for local workers (Fig. 9).

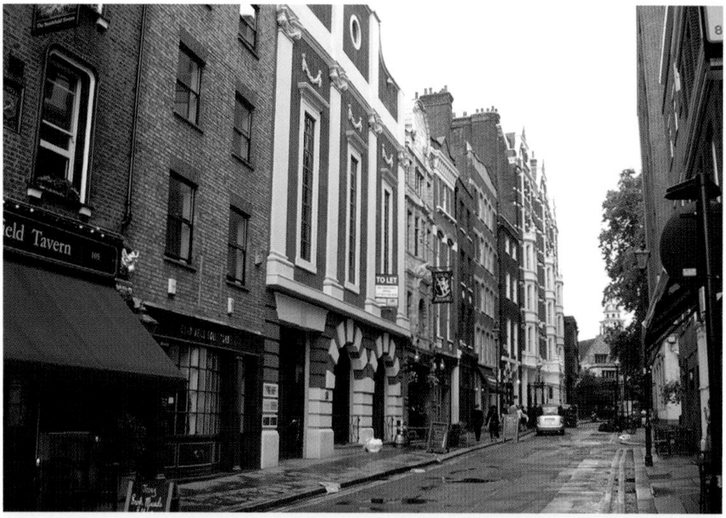

The Great Fire of London, 1666, destroyed many houses on Fleet Street but these were rapidly rebuilt following the same architectural design and layout. Local trades included watch making, publishing, gin distilling and furniture making as well as those that flourished in a supplementary role to the market, such as butchers and bacon-smokers.

Figure 9 Charterhouse Street, Farringdon
(Greg Dunlap, cc-by-sa/2.0 https://www.flickr.com/photos/heyrocker/3737914864)

Hatton Garden continued to operate as a centre for jewellery production. In the mid-19th century, the scale of development rapidly altered with the introduction of the Metropolitan Railway at Farringdon station in 1863 as well as the earlier King's Cross Station in 1850. Slums were cleared and new roads were constructed, increasing the areas connections to additional parts of the City. A new market building was constructed at Smithfields and by the early 20th century, the area's residential capacity began to fall, being superseded by small scale industries. This has continued, with Clerkenwell having been designated as 'Use Class', ensuring new developments were for light industries and commerce only. Today, following the introduction of clean air policies, the closure of the gin distillery and reduction of the meat markets, it has transformed into an area rich in professional services such as leisure and entertainment, design and media.

London pre-industrial sites (1066–*c*. 1750)

Billingsgate derives its name from 'Blynesgate' or 'Byllynsgate', referring to the original watergate on the Thames where goods were landed. Construction developments took place in the 9th century under Alfred the Great creating new

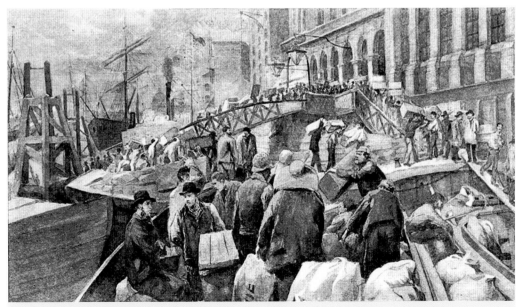

Figure 10 Billingsgate Fish Market, from *Sketches of England by a Foreign Artist* by Mons Myrbach, 1891
(British Library, Public Domain)

wharves and waterside markets selling fish, grain, salt and timber, establishing it as a major port from the late Saxon period. Due to its prominence as a location for imports in the medieval period, the area was filled with grocery businesses, dealing in spices, medicines, dyes, as well as exotic foodstuffs such as pepper, sugar, figs, ginger, rice and dates. 'Pepperers', as they were formerly known formed an association in the late 12th century and subsequently a Grocer's Guild in the 14th century. During the later medieval period, the Billingsgate market area expanded and specialised, becoming the well-known fish market it is today by about 1650 (Fig. 10). Throughout the pre-Industrial period, Billingsgate was a hub of commercial and international mercantile activity in the City.

St Mary Graces, Royal Mint, East Smithfield has a long affinity with religious orders. East Smithfield was first given to the church of the Holy Trinity within Aldgate in 1115 by Henry I. One area of land was occupied, however, by Geoffrey de Mandeville, who had cultivated a vineyard and rejected calls to vacate the site. The Hospital of St Katherine was founded here in 1148. The site was later granted to the Cistercian order in 1350 and the Abbey of St Mary Graces, also known as Eastminster (Fig. 11),

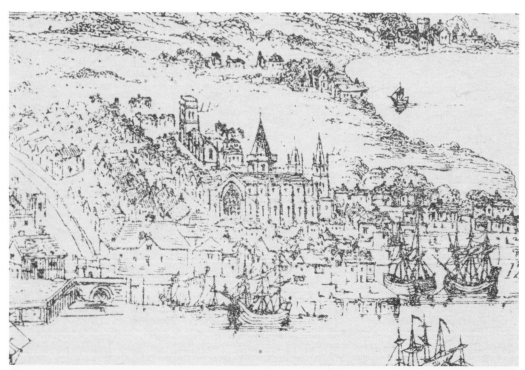

Figure 11 The Abbey of St Mary de Graces (Eastminster), from *A View of London, Westminster and Southwark 1543* by Wyngaerde
(© Museum of London)

was the last Cistercian foundation in Britain. It became the third wealthiest such establishment in England.

The area consisted of open fields that were used during the Black Death in the mid-14th century to create substantial emergency burial grounds. Following the dissolution of the priory in 1538–9, the Hospital of St Katherine was maintained as a protestant house, with houses and a brewery being built in the precinct. Since its wharves were outside the City, St Katherine's Quay was used for unloading foreign ships, predominantly from Holland, which were not allowed to dock in the City itself. The area took on a cosmopolitan character with many people from France and beyond settling here. St Katherine's became renowned for its brewhouses.

Non-metropolitan pre-industrial sites (1066–*c.* 1750)

Hereford was an important medieval town, or 'shire' town, and thought to have been founded as a market around AD 958. The market, well attended by people from all over the neighbouring counties, provided the main source of wealth for building of the Cathedral (Fig. 12). This then functioned as a money-generating centre of pilgrimage for the city, where devotees came to visit the shrines of St Ethelbert and St Thomas Cantilupe. A motte and bailey castle was also built here to defend The Marches, a tract of land along the border between England and Wales subject to constant skirmishes. Given its Royal ownership, much of the town's development involved planned building work. The construction of the Cathedral and castle were accompanied by large scale deforestation and land clearance to accommodate its new owners and tenants. The history of the town was tumultuous during the 12th century when it was besieged by Stephen and Matilda. The arable farmlands were maintained in an open field system but climate change

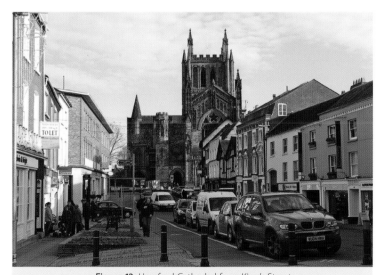

Figure 12 Hereford Cathedral from King's Street
(David Merrett, cc-by/2.0, https://www.flickr.com/photos/davehamster/5269161236)

and famines, as in many areas of Britain, took their toll as well as the Black Death in 1349. The situation was further aggravated by pastoral enclosure of its agricultural fields. However, the resulting wool trade flourished in the 14th century, allowing an extensive new phase of building work at the Cathedral as well as at several churches. A grammar school was also founded on the proceeds. Although several of the more rural settlements in the county declined and were abandoned, Hereford maintained its economy through the industries of wool making and leather working and continued to thrive.

These trades were still active throughout the 19th century and even until very recently, the city has predominantly retained its rural 'market town' character, with little industry involving manufacture for export. Hereford has recently seen a number of regeneration projects, including the amalgamation of its previous health care services into one much larger hospital, costing £60 million, and the relocation of the historic cattle market to a site on the outskirts of the City following the 2001 foot-and-mouth outbreak, which led to a significant decline in trade.

Non-metropolitan pre-industrial and industrial sites (1066–1900)

Barton-upon-Humber, originally called 'Beretun', or Barley Town was a major settlement in the Anglo-Saxon period and in 1086 was recorded as having a church, a market, two mills and a ferry, being populated by about 1000 people. Its size and importance were due to its function as the main port of north Lincolnshire through which wines, fish, peas, wool, hide and grains were traded. Edward I founded 'Kingstown upon Hull' in 1293 on the opposite bank to the north but Barton continued to grow due to its rich agricultural lands. In 1359, the town provided eight ships and 121 men for Edward III's expedition to France, which was later followed by more sea-bound expeditions in the English Civil and Napoleonic wars. During the early Industrial period enclosure rapidly led to a reorganisation of the local fields and roads and the local economy correspondingly shifted from one that was almost completely agricultural to involving manufacture, especially of brick and tile (Fig. 13) but also rope making using locally grown raw materials, candle making, cycle manufacture, engineering, malting and ship building.

Shipping merchants expanded their trade networks to Greenland for whaling and to the West Indies in addition to maintaining a local trade for importing coal and exporting bricks. At least six brick built mills had appeared by 1800 that were eventually converted from wind to steam or oil power. Thatch cottages were replaced by brick houses during the late 18th and 19th centuries. The population expanded rapidly from 1709 people in 1801 to 5671 people in 1901, and there were numerous prospering trades located along Barton's wharfs. Local amenities were added to the town during this time, including transport infrastructure, sports clubs and a police station. During the 20th century the town unfortunately endured the decline of many previously important local trades but commuting has been made possible through the construction Humber Bridge and the town has gradually started to recover.

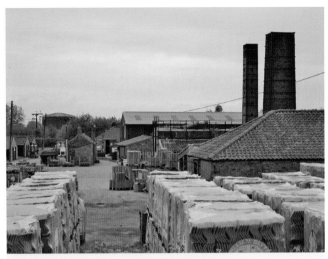

Figure 13 Hoe Hill Tilery, Barton-upon-Humber, established in 1840 by William Blythe, now the only yard working in Barton

Stratford-upon-Avon is an ancient town that was part of an estate held by the Church of Worcester as early as the 7th century. The older part of the town retains its original layout based on three parallel streets and three streets perpendicular to the river (Fig. 14). The majority of the houses were located on these central streets next to fairly open, rural grounds with barns and closes. Two watercourses still ran through the town until 1804, which were used to power a mill. Buildings were of timber construction, though some of these were replaced after a number of fires, two particularly disastrous conflagrations in 1594 and 1595 having destroyed 200 houses. Subsequently, thatched roofs were banned and tiles were used for residential properties, though barns and outbuildings close by were still thatched. Still under the threat of fire, the first fire engine was introduced to Stratford in 1684 and a second in 1694.

Although the River Avon had been made navigable up to Stratford by 1636, the town did not expand until the 19th century when the canal was completed and the ability to transport goods into and out of the centre of town was achieved. From the 1830s, some industry then started to develop but this was generally quite slow paced. A large part of the local economy still depended on its rural subsistence. By virtue of its location on the main roads across the county, leading to major towns such as

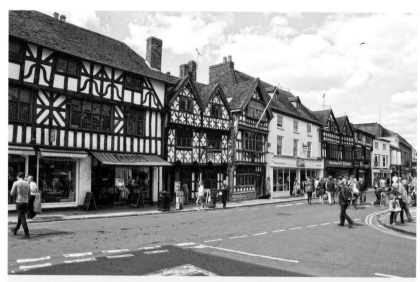

Figure 14 The High Street, Stratford-upon-Avon, looking from the junction with Sheep Street.
(cc-by-sa/2.0 - © Lewis Clarke - geograph.org.uk/p/3969615)

Oxford and Birmingham, the local horse fair, founded in the mid-17th century, and the sheep market, dating to 1265, continued to be highly successful. Related local trades, such as glovers and sellers of butter, cheese and meats, were supplemented by manufacturing industries such as ironmongers, nailers, collar makers, braziers and pewterers and rope makers. The town had a brick kiln, coal yard and storehouse and additionally supported a Baker's Company, a Faculty of Tailors and a malting industry. Following the increased traffic in the Industrial period some older streets were demolished to make way for wider roads and the coaching industry became important to the town with at least 24 coaches a day passing through Stratford heading to London, Birmingham, Shrewsbury and Holyhead in 1817. The first gas works were established in 1834 and Stratford continued to be an important distribution point for coal throughout Staffordshire. Following the decline of such local industries with the introduction of green legislation, Stratford today is a major tourist attraction as the birthplace of William Shakespeare and continues to be an important strategic location for logistics-based businesses.

Wharram Percy, in Yorkshire, is today considered as a 'deserted medieval village' forming a heritage site, with only the Church and earthworks remaining of the village (Fig. 15). However, the site was once a prospering medieval village, situated in about 8500 acres (*c.* 3440 ha) of farm and pasture land, which was occupied for over 600

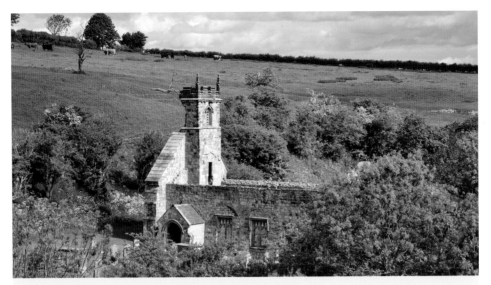

Figure 15 Wharram Percy Church

years from the late Anglo-Saxon period. Originally the village comprised two Manors, one North and one South but the South Manor was subsequently demolished while the North Manor was improved. At this time, two more rows of cottages were built, leading to total of about 40 houses. A small hunting park was established by around 1320. The village was largely self-sufficient, with in-house meat, leather and wool production as well as corn milling, though some items found during excavation of the site originate from the Mediterranean and France. There were raids by the Scots in 1319–1322 and this led to the devastation of neighbouring Thixendale, when seven farmsteads were raised to the ground by fire. At this point, the population began to decline and two-thirds of the land went uncultivated while houses stood empty and the watermills went unused. There was a short period of recovery but the Black Death plague of 1348 led to a reduction of the general population, resulting in a shortage of labourers and an increase in wages demanded by them.

The need for higher incomes led to the turning over of arable land to pasture to profit from increasing wool prices but this was disastrous for arable farmers and many villages like Wharram Percy went into terminal decline. Four families were evicted from Wharram in about 1500 and their houses were pulled down. Only a handful of shepherds remained and the last arable plots were converted to pasture in 1527. The village formally ceased to exist in 1636 and the area became a farmstead. The last burial in the Churchyard took place in 1906.

Non-metropolitan industrial sites (*c.* 1750–1900)

Brentford: although Brentford is now an area in outer London, near Ealing, Hanwell and Isleworth, for most of its history it has been an independent satellite town located outside the City in a comparatively rural setting. In 1306, under the aegis of the Abbess and nuns of St Helens, Bishopgate at Boston Manor, a license for a fair and a market was granted to the settlement. Brentford was a typical medieval town with local production of goods such as bricks and timber and being furnished with a brew-house, wharves onto the river and public houses with a bowling alley. It was only one of three towns marked on a map in the west London area in 1595 and was visited by Pocahontas in 1616. The settlement actually comprised Old Brentford and New Brentford, the latter seemingly being the more recent and wealthier part of town. Over the course of the 17th century parcels of land were sold for development. Old cottages were demolished for the construction of a market house in 1666, which was set in extended grounds, for the expanding trade in sheep and pigs. In 1711 records show that horticulture was starting to become prominent in the

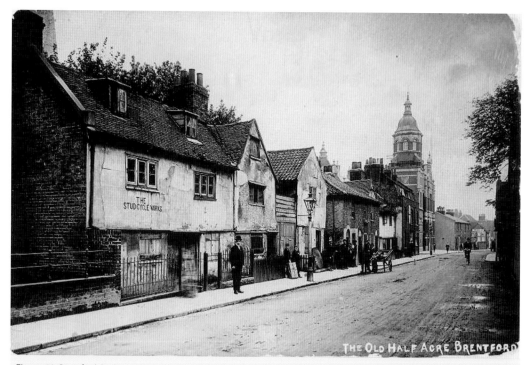

Figure 16 Brentford, looking south down Half Acre towards the junction with the High Street. The Stud Cycle Works are advertised on the building on the left. The ornate building further on is the Vestry Hall, built 1900

(© Howard Webb, with permission of The Brentford High Street Project, www.bhsproject.co.uk)

local economy and land was being used to grow mulberries, apples, cherries, asparagus and strawberries to supply the London market. By 1745 orchards and market gardens are clearly identifiable on maps encompassed by open fields, home to large estates at Syon, Osterley, Boston and Gunnersby. Roads were woefully poor, the High Street having been described in the *Gentleman's Magazine* in 1754 as the worst public road in Europe, despite continuing and increasing traffic to Bath and London. The town continued to increase in size and by 1793, its industries comprised flour milling, malt distilling, brewing, brick making, pottery, turpentine and soap making. Fishing was also an important local source of income but this had declined by 1845.

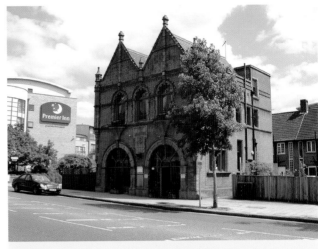

Figure 17 Old Fire Station, Brentford, surrounded by modern urban development

(Maxwell Hamilton, cc-by/2.0, https://www.flickr.com/photos/mualphachi/3795550315)

However, market gardening continued to flourish. Hugh Ronalds, a local landowner, was said in 1829 to have been producing 300 different varieties of apples and supplied 14,000 shrubs to Kensal Green cemetery, probably transported along the canal, where the Grand Junction Waterworks opened at Kew Bridge in 1835. Despite the fact that landowners were thriving, the town's population was beset with poverty from the 19th century and many were still living in old, run-down housing (Fig. 16). In 1873, the *Brentford Advertiser* described it as the filthiest place in England. In 1875, Old and New Brentford as well as Brentford End were amalgamated and its increased urbanisation, including the introduction of trams, trains, a fire station (Fig. 17), swimming baths, sports clubs and a library between 1883 and 1901, eventually saw it engulfed by the encroaching suburbs of outer London.

Fewston is a remote parish in the West Riding of Yorkshire which, in the early medieval period, actually consisted of two separate settlements called 'Fostune' (Fewston) and Bestham (Beeston), the latter of which eventually became part of the former. Fewston was a township that was part of a wider area of hunting ground, including three further townships, set aside for Royalty and, therefore, land use was restricted. Although some enclosure and ploughing were later allowed, this was still limited to local residents and forest managers. The population increased and cottage industries sprang up while the land was still farmed. Stone quarrying, iron working and coal mining were part of the local industries. In 1526 a license was granted to Fewston for processing wool at a fulling mill. A combination of the increasing encroachment onto the Royal Estate by local landowners and the enclosure of land for sheep pasture in 1755 ensured that this industry then flourished in the village. The old fulling mill was converted to a corn mill while a massive new mill called West House (Fig. 18) was constructed in 1797 using the river Washburn to spin flax and later weave linen.

The processes became increasingly mechanised but cheap labour from the local poorer towns in the area, in addition to apprentice boys and girls brought from London, were also used to work the mill, often working 13 hour days. Extensive engineering took place to create the required new dams needed but a decline in trade shortly afterwards meant that the mill owners became bankrupt in 1844. It later reopened in 1861 as a much smaller silk mill business but closed only 3 years later. The demand for water in Leeds was met by the construction of Fewston Reservoir in 1874, as well as a number of other local reservoirs, that required the demolition of local houses and buildings. Fewston Mill was demolished and West House Mill followed in 1877. The reservoir, opened in 1879, has a capacity of 3.5 million cubic metres and a circumference of 3.7 miles (5.45 km). At its peak, Fewston had approximately 850 inhabitants but, following the successive failures of the mill and the imposition of the expansive reservoir, the size of the local population declined and today remains very small, at only 182 people.

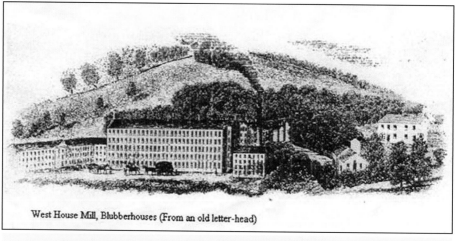

West House Mill, Blubberhouses (From an old letter-head)

Figure 18 Old letter heading detailing West House Mill, Blubberhouses, Fewston
(Church of England http://www.fewstonwithblubberhouses.org.uk/our-churches/fewston-church/parish-of-fewston/)

North Shields was originally a fishing port under the control of Tynemouth Priory in the 13th century and its name stems from the 'shiels' or turf huts the fishermen lived in at Pow Burn, or Fish Quay as it is today. After the local marshlands were drained, the settlement of three huts eventually grew to 200 houses and included mills, taverns, bake houses, the Fish Quay and a brewery. Most houses had their own quays and trade via the sea thrived until Edward I demanded fees and limited trade. However, the town started to flourish once more following transfer of the lands to the Earl of Northumberland in 1539. While the region between Tynemouth and South Shields is rich in coal and most of the local industries were heavily based on mining, North Shields continued with its substantial fishing industry. Clifford's Fort was constructed in 1672 to defend the town from press-gang raids. In 1796, 250 mechanics and sailors were press-ganged to serve in the Royal Navy, despite the defence of local troops.

The town was huddled around the quays and much of the housing consisted of tightly packed narrow fronted, tall residences that were cramped and had no sanitation or amenities. North Shields was a busy urban centre, however, with many trades and amenities, such as public houses, coffee houses, dance houses, bakers and mast makers, rope makers and clothes dealers. Local industry focused on the docks also featured five iron foundries, a large tannery, two salt works, a pottery and steam mills for grinding corn. In 1830, as the town expanded, the first steamships began to operate the North and South Shields Ferry Company and in 1858 steamers commenced trading between North Shields and the Black Sea. Goods included flour, biscuits, sugar, peas, beans rice, salted fish, hams, teas, butter and lard. 'Woodgers Exporters' sent 20,000,000 kippers annually to London and country markets. The shipping trade had doubled as early as 1762 and with this wealthy shipping merchants, as well as doctors and lawyers, settled in the town and began to construct more lavish housing in Dockwray Square and Northumberland Square, away from the crowded harbour area, up on the higher ground beyond (Fig. 19). In 1827 waggonways

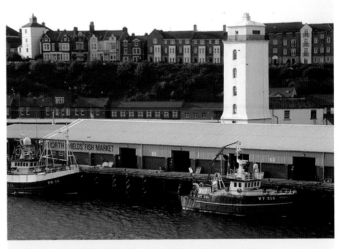

Figure 19 The Fish Market, North Shields.
(cc-by-sa/2.0 - © Colin Smith - geograph.org.uk/p/3136250)

for transporting coal from Whitley colliery to the colliers' brigs at the Quays were constructed and in 1857, North Shields was also connected to the railway.

As the ship trade declined, the town started to experience an economic downturn. Some of the previously more comfortable housing was turned into tenements and became slums. In 1956, the east end of North Shields was declared unfit for human habitation and Dockwray Square was demolished. With many of the local major employers ceasing to trade, North Shields has experienced some difficult times including the Meadow Well riots. However, in 1992, a government regeneration scheme of £37.5 million commenced with redevelopment of the abandoned Albert Edward docks. Public amenities including sports facilities were upgraded, Fish Quay saw regeneration through the construction of luxury apartments and the site of the former Smith's Docks is currently being redeveloped by *Places for People*.

Swinton, Salford: Until 1865 Swinton was a small hamlet in the township of Worsley, near Eccles, now part of greater Manchester. The name Swinton is derived from the Old English 'Swynton' meaning 'swine town'. It was part of the lands of Whalley Abbey and the Knights Hospitaller, generating incomes from farming and hand-loom weaving. Swinton was also an important staging post along the principal road from Manchester to Lancaster. The town expanded in the Industrial Period due to its proximity to coal fields, which were the source of fuel for the nearby brick making factories and cotton mills. By the mid-19th century, Swinton had become a well-established mill town surrounded by newly constructed transport infrastructure, factories and brickworks. However, its location was still relatively rural. The implementation of mass manufacturing led to a lot of poverty for the local population working in traditional trades, who arranged a 'Blanketeers' Demonstration in 1817 and marched to London in protest. The economic situation worsened with the cotton famine, especially between 1862 and 1865 when poor relief was being continually sought in the town. Some benefits of industrialisation were felt in the town though, with the opening of the Swinton Industrial School to aid children in poorer families, which remained open until the 1920s, along with Sunday Schools and libraries. In 1868, the Manchester Corporation finally finished introducing the necessary infrastructure to pipe clean water into the town and at the same time, Swinton's streets were lit by gaslights (Fig. 20). Victoria Park was also opened in 1897 to provide an open public space.

The town by this time was continuing to expand but also being further encroached on by its neighbouring districts in Salford, ending its separation by open fields from local settlements. Today, Swinton is largely a commuter town due to its connection

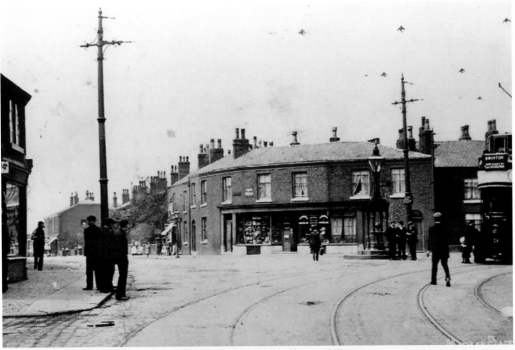

Figure 20 Swinton Market Place, *c.* 1905
(Public domain)

to the East Lancashire Road, Britain's first intercity highway, allowing easy access to Manchester city centre.

Upton-upon-Severn, Worcestershire, is located on what was an important crossing site of the River Severn from the Welsh border to the Avon Valley and until the latter half of the 20th century, provided the only bridge across the river between Worcester and Tewkesbury. The route was used as a drove for cattle and sheep from the Welsh to English markets. Maintaining the bridge there over time has been a continual occupation, upgrading the wooden bridge, thought to be present from about 1480, to a stone bridge shortly after and repairing the bridge again in 1852 after it was eroded by a great flood, which again was to be replaced in 1940 by the present bridge. Keeping the river free for access has also proved to be a continual struggle due to the build-up of a shoal which, in 1849, was reported to have grounded 200–300 sailing vessels at a time. The town thrived with a market and numerous fairs, with the local economy predominantly based on crop farming and animal husbandry.

Fishing was also a major local economic source to the extent that, in 1613, a

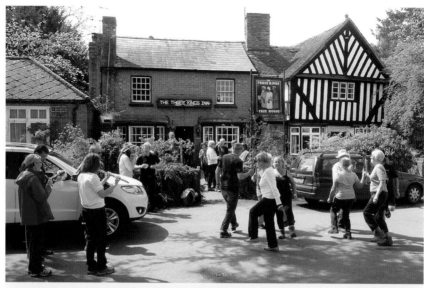

Figure 21 *Upton-upon-Severn Folk Festival 2015*

petition was submitted against the Upton fishermen for exhausting fish stocks in the whole river. The area was heavily involved in the English Civil War in 1651 but Upton was prosperous during the Industrial Revolution, when new Georgian housing was constructed, though the town retained its traditional market town character (Fig. 21). Upton suffered numerous periods of flooding throughout its history and flood defence work has continued up to the present day in order to prevent the lower lying areas of the town being inundated by flood water as they were in the past (Fig. 22). Upton continues to thrive as a small market town of independent retailers and service providers.

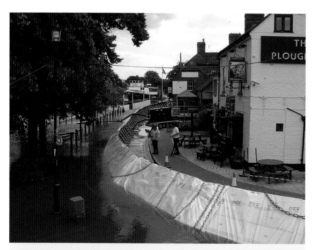

Figure 22 The Plough Inn at Upton-upon-Severn. Protected from Flooding, June 2007

Table 1 London and non-metropolitan sites from the pre-Industrial and Industrial periods selected for research project with total numbers of individuals in each group radiographed and social status only for London Industrial

Date range	Site name	Site code	No. individuals radiographed	Period	Social status London Industrial*
1450–1666	Billingsgate, London	BIG82	29	Pre-Industrial	–
1569–1714	Broadgate, London	LSS85	61	Pre-Industrial	–
1348–1350	East Smithfield, London	MIN86	12	Pre-Industrial	–
1350–1539	St Mary Graces, London	NBR98	8	Pre-Industrial	–
1120–1539	St Mary Spital, London	SRP98	399	Pre-Industrial	–
1840–1855	Bethnal Green, London	PGV10	201	Industrial	Low Status
1816–1853	Bow Baptists, London	BBP07/PAY05	127	Industrial	Low Status
1712–1842	Chelsea Old Church, London	OCU00	35	Industrial	High Status
c. 1812–1853	Mare Street, Hackney, London	MRH14	145	Industrial	High Status
c. 1830–1850	New Covent Garden, Nine Elms, London	NNE16	23	Industrial	–
1750–1852	St Bride's Crypt, London	SB79	175	Industrial	High Status
1770–1849	St Bride's Lower Churchyard, London	FAO90	136	Industrial	Low Status
950–1500	Barton upon Humber	BH81 (Phase C & D medieval)	134	Pre-Industrial	–
1140–1500	Hereford Cathedral	HE93a	50	Pre-Industrial	–
1322–1650	Holy Trinity Stratford	P4442 Phase 1–3	48	Pre-Industrial	–
950–1540	Wharram Percy	WPMed	127	Pre-Industrial	–
c. 1700–1855	Barton upon Humber	BH81 (Phase A & B post- medieval)	189	Industrial	–
1828–1868	Brentford	HHS14	108	Industrial	–
1710–1833	Coach Lane, North Shields	COL10	88	Industrial	–
1700–1896	Fewston, West Yorkshire	SLF09	24	Industrial	–
c. 1750–1887	Holy Trinity Stratford	P4442	33	Industrial	–
1820–1900	Swinton, Salford	SWC12	50	Industrial	–
1836–1866	Upton-upon-Severn, Worcestershire	WSM43246	10	Industrial	–
c. 1700–1850	Wharram Percy	WPPMED	29	Industrial	–

(* based on burial location/type and burial furnishings)

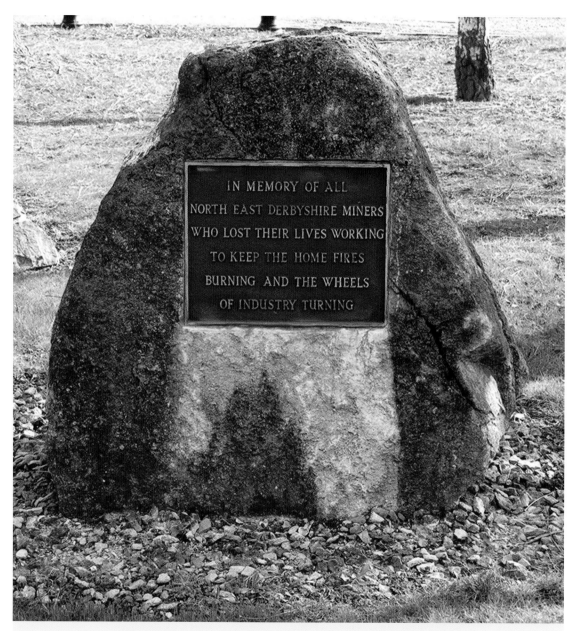

Figure 23 Memorial to north-east Derbyshire miners who lost their lives at work

1

Occupational hazards and sporting catastrophes

It's a bit funny but we are a dying breed paying homage to the already dead. Well we are, there are none of us to follow...People of Swinton and Pendlebury, please tell your children about us, tell them about those who have gone before, of the blood, sweat and tears they shed in order to make this a better place, take them on the heritage trail so thoughtfully provided by your council. The mining families of the past fought, suffered and died for the rights we now enjoy, please don't let them down.

Brian, father of Adam Stott (336), the last miner to die at Agecroft Colliery, Swinton. 29 May 2016

At 9.20am on Thursday 18 June 1885, for some, time stood still. A huge explosion occurred at Clifton Hall Colliery, near Swinton, Salford that could be felt at a distance of half a mile (0.8 km). In total, 178 men and boys were killed through injuries, burns, drowning or by the effects of 'afterdamp' (carbon monoxide poisoning). The bodies of the miners were buried at numerous churchyards and burial grounds in the locality, including the Jane Lane burial ground, which was subject to commercial development in 2013, some 130 years later. The human remains in the burial ground pre-dating 1900 were not cleared away but instead were exhumed and recorded by archaeologists prior to reburial in Swinton cemetery, forming one of our study groups for this project. Through this process the remains of some of the victims of the Clifton Hall Colliery disaster were identified and its history once more brought to light. Unfortunately, incidents like these were all too common during this period, a time of industrial accidents on an industrial scale. Construction projects were implemented at a furious rate during the Victorian period and were notoriously dangerous. It has been calculated, for example, that three labourers died for every mile of rail track laid in the UK. Mortality rates were even higher for the railway tunnellers. Thirty-two labourers were killed and at least 140 seriously injured while working on the Woodhead Tunnel between Manchester and Sheffield, which runs for 3 miles (4.8 km). That's one death plus 4–5 serious injuries for every 495 ft or 150 m.

Accidents, of course, were not just restricted to the work-place. Cities like London were energetic places of hustle and bustle, people constantly on the go, with no time to waste and ever in haste. The lack of regular maintenance checks and health and safety regulations meant that the potential for danger lurked on every corner and not only in the towns; roads everywhere were a source of constant threat, especially with the use of horse-drawn carts on pot-holed tracks. Road safety was not a concept and nor was there any lawful responsibility on the part of the builders of temporary constructions, machines or contraptions, which many people used in the home or as part of recreation on a daily basis. Some injuries, of course, were also sustained through acts of violence resulting from wars, domestic abuse, or 'Peaky Blinders' style rival gang brutality. Others were caused by common sporting activities such as horse riding, boxing or shooting. The recording of traumatic injuries in skeletal remains by archaeologists, supplemented by historic accounts of events happening at the time, gives us a very stark reminder of the scale of unfortunate misdemeanours and human disasters that occurred in the past and how this compares with our heavily safety-regulated living environments today.

London is nowadays associated with high levels of accidents and violence on account of the high population density and sheer volume of vehicular traffic in the City. Was this also the case in the past? Was life in the City really more hazardous compared to more rural settings? How did accidents and trauma impact upon our bodies in the past and was this different according to where we lived?

Pre-industrial lifestyles and trauma risk

Trauma is predominantly influenced by the environment in which we live and work, and the medieval period in Britain was no exception. During this time the country was predominantly agricultural and jobs were labour intensive. For many, food production, brewing and farming were day-in, day-out tasks of hard, manual labour. This would have extended to the maintenance and repairs of their own houses, barns or other property. Occupational hazards, then, were surprisingly common, even within rural settings.

Some of the more risky environments would have been experienced by the raft of tradesmen specialising in jobs that were more industrial in nature, such as carpentry, candle making, milling, brick and tile production, quarrying, mining, cloth making, smelting and blacksmithing (Fig. 24). As the population grew throughout the medieval period not only did the agricultural economy intensify, with more and more land cleared for crop growing, but also technologies involving the production of foods, materials and transport advanced. The 6500 turnable mills already in existence in England in 1086, as documented in *Domesday Book*, were quickly superseded by vertical windmills, the earliest of which in Europe is thought to date to 1185, located in the former village of Weedley in Yorkshire, overlooking the Humber Estuary. The wide-ranging major technological advances and inventions in medieval Europe from the 12th century led to the mechanisation of many production processes, although these industries were still in their infancies compared to the vast scale of mass production experienced from 1750 onwards in England.

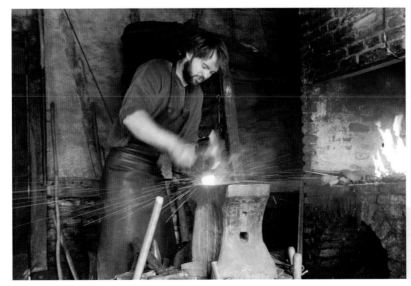

Figure 24 Recreating medieval blacksmithing.

(Hans Splinter, cc-by-nd/2.0, https://www.flickr.com/photos/archeon/10493442664)

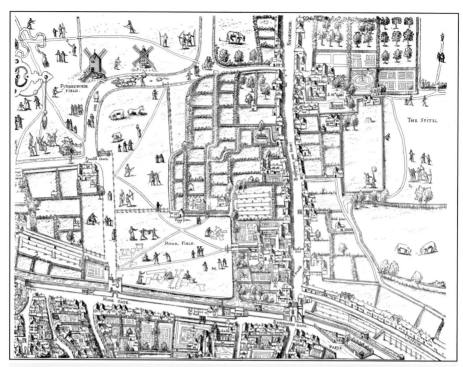

Figure 25 Copperplate map 1559, Frans Franken, section showing Moorfields and The Spital

(© Museum of London)

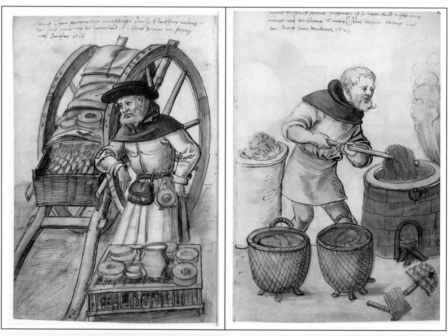

Figure 26 Cheese merchant at market and textile dyer

(Paul K. cc-by/2.0, https://www.flickr.com/photos/bibliodyssey/albums/72157610727752183)

Towns, and even cities such as London, were much smaller and less densely populated than today. Many areas in the City during the medieval period, such as Nine Elms, Bow, Hackney, Bethnal Green, Chelsea and Spitalfields, were small hamlets, villages or bases for religious houses, surrounded by open greenfields used for market gardening, agriculture and meadowland (Fig. 25).

Over time, as trade between settlements grew and more goods were transported by land and by river, the market economy developed (Fig. 26). Markets in towns flourished, and those in the City such as Billingsgate, where originally many goods such as corn, coal, iron, salt pottery and fish could be purchased, eventually specialised; Billingsgate for example became the world famous fish market.

The market wealth generated led to the construction of an increasing number of prestigious large stone buildings, in particular, strongholds and cathedrals, as well as bridges. The building of Westminster Abbey, completed in 1066, and West Minster Hall, started in 1097, not only consolidated the position of William the Conqueror as the King of England but also London's status as the political and mercantile centre of the country. The City's higher status and clerical role led to the creation of many bureaucratic and professional occupations. The construction trade, in contrast, was very hazardous, with little to protect workers from substantial falls and injuries (Fig. 27).

Written accounts at St Paul's Cathedral, dating to the time of Sir Christopher Wren's construction from 1675, record compensation payments to the widows of builders who died from falls at the site. Additionally, analysis of the medieval human remains from Hereford Cathedral, carried out by the University of Bradford, revealed a high number of fractures, including multiple injuries and crush fractures among males, likely related to the contemporary building works in the city of the Cathedral and the castle, although these were healed fractures,

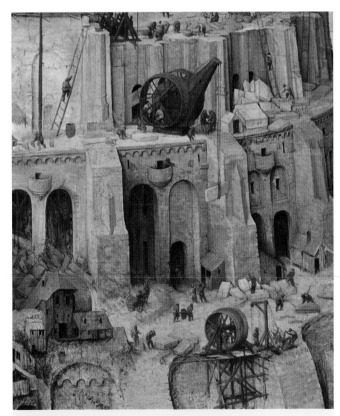

Figure 27 Bruegel's Tower of Babel, detailing stone construction and use of the treadmill crane

(rpi virtuell, cc-by/2.0, https://www.flickr.com/photos/84132860@N03/7702914260)

indicating that the injuries sustained were not fatal.

Also present at Hereford Cathedral, as found elsewhere such as at Barton-upon-Humber, Wharram Percy and in London, were several examples of sharp force cranial trauma inflicted through violent assaults using bladed weapons (Fig. 28).

Warfare throughout the country was almost endemic and a significant number of the medieval male population would have taken part in armed combat (Fig. 29). In fact, medieval London was founded by a siege on the City in 1066 led by William the Conqueror, 'causing no little mourning to the City because of the very many deaths of her own sons and citizens' according to the Norman chronicler, William of Jumieges. Important roles within the fighting forces included archers, bowmen, pikemen and spearmen. Carrying sharp

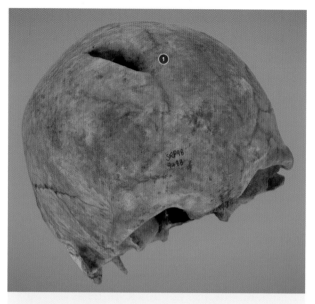

Figure 28 3D model of healed sharp force cranial trauma, (1). young adult male, pre-Industrial London

(SRP98 9488) 3D models available to view at https://sketchfab.com/jbekvalac

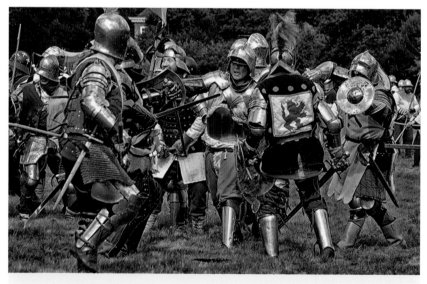

Figure 29 Medieval battle re-enactment, Herstmonceux Castle, Sussex

(Vicki Burton, cc-by-sa/2.0, https://www.flickr.com/photos/vicki_burton)

bladed weapons such as knives was an everyday norm.

Sports were another source of potential injury. Medieval or mob football (Fig. 30) involved opposing teams of large crowds of men from neighbouring towns rampaging through the streets to get a ball, made from an inflated pig's bladder, to the markers at one end of the town. Any means could be used, as long as it avoided manslaughter or murder! The game is still played today in Ashbourne, Derbyshire where it is known as Royal Shrovetide Football (Fig. 31).

Unfortunately, mob football was so violent in the past that accidental deaths and injuries, sometimes involving knives, sheathed or otherwise, were frequent enough to warrant Nicholas de Farndone, the mayor of the City of London, banning football in 1314. Furthermore, Edward III also issued a decree in 1363 prohibiting 'stone, wood and iron throwing, handball, football or hockey; coursing, cockfighting, or other such idle games' under penalty of imprisonment. As witnessed by William Fitz Stephen *c.* 1173, ice skating (Fig. 32) on frozen rivers and marshes in London was also very popular. Winter games included a chain of people dragging another person seated on a chair along the ice, usually falling onto their faces during the process, and also pole-vaulting over the icy surface. This often involved two people running at each other and vaulting simultaneously, the velocity of their entangled fall commonly leading to broken arms and legs.

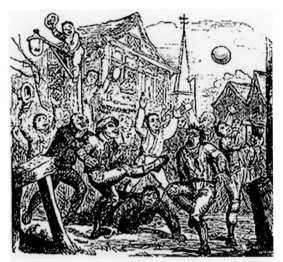

Figure 30 A mob football match played at Crowe Street, London 1721

(public domain, PD-Art (PD UK), https://commons.wikimedia.org/wiki/File:Mobfooty.jpg)

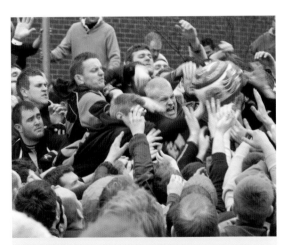

Figure 31 The Royal Shrovetide Football at Ashbourne

(Will de Freitas, cc-by-nd/2.0, https://www.flickr.com/photos/ninjawil/6775534742/in/photostream/)

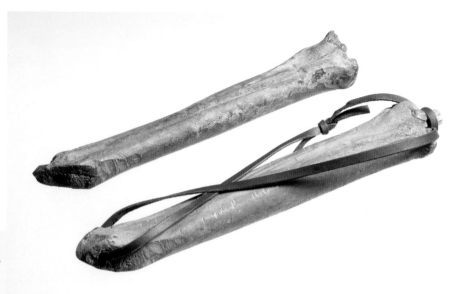

Trauma and lifestyles in rural small towns in the Industrial period

By the Industrial period, the population was growing fast and urbanisation intensifying. It is estimated that, in 1750, only about 15% of the population lived in towns whereas by 1900 the proportion of urban dwellers had risen substantially to 85%. Urban areas quickly became crammed with overcrowded housing, workshops, warehouses and traffic. However, this was not the case everywhere. The demand for water and transportation following the swell of migration to the rapidly expanding cities led to major land redevelopment. Construction projects and engineering feats were very often at the cost of rural towns and villages. The building of the reservoir in 1874 at Fewston in West

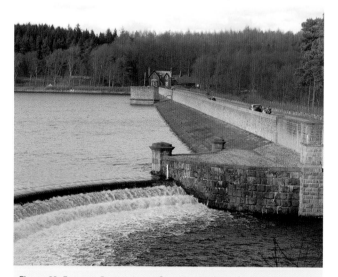

Figure 33 Fewston Reservoir overflow, West Riding of Yorkshire

Yorkshire (Fig. 33), for example, provided a source of water for Leeds but simultaneously led to the demolition of extensive local mills, which in former days had been the nucleus of the local economy and settlement.

Many rural villages like Wharram Percy in East Yorkshire went into decline and were abandoned after the medieval period following a switch of land use from agriculture to pasture to exploit the rising export prices of wool from the late 15th century (Fig. 34). Sheep farming had become a lucrative business and tenant farmers were evicted over a number of years, leading to its eventual abandonment. Thomas More, commenting on the issue at the time, wrote:

> The increase in pasture, by which your sheep, which are naturally mild and easily kept in order, may now be said to devour men, and unpeople, not only villages, but towns; for whenever it is found that the sheep of any soil yield a softer and richer wool than ordinary, there the nobility and gentry, and even those holy men the abbots, not contented with the old rents which their farms yielded, not thinking it enough that they, living at their ease, do no good to the public, resolve to do it hurt instead of good. (*Utopia*, 1516)

This was compounded by the *Enclosure Acts* from the early 18th century that aimed to fence off and reorganise field systems in order to make them more productive for agriculture and pasture. Larger plots allowed for mechanised, more intensive

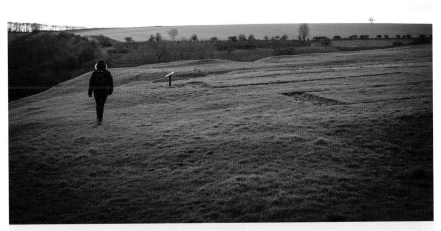

Figure 34 Earthworks from the deserted medieval village at Wharram Percy
(Dr Colleen Morgan, cc-by/2.0, https://www.flickr.com/photos/colleenmorgan/)

production methods. However, this resulted in an obliteration of what had previously been common land, so that smaller tenant holders reliant on common land were forced out. They either became dependent on wealthier landowners for jobs or had to migrate and take factory work in the towns and cities. As with many villages and towns, the long term fate of remote and seemingly isolated places, like Wharram Percy and Fewston, was dependent upon economic forces that were tied to the restructuring of the nation's infrastructure to meet the demands of global markets and the industrial boom.

Many rural towns did continue to thrive during the Industrial period, on either agricultural and pastoral economies such as Upton-on-Severn and Stratford-upon-Avon, as satellite towns to industrialised cities, such as Swinton or Brentford, or as ports and harbours such as North Shields and Barton-upon-Humber. However, life remained physically laborious for the inhabitants. Many daily tasks were still manual and quite often dangerous, which we see skeletal evidence for. One old adult male SK[8010] from Upton-on-Severn, for example, had suffered a serious fracture to the left ankle. As a result of the injury, the whole ankle had been flattened and remodelled, with atrophy or thinning of the foot bones from its subsequent disuse (see Fig. 35). This

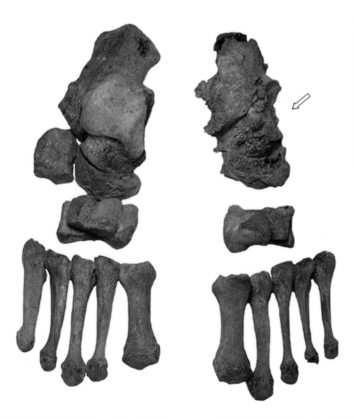

Figure 35 Impact fracture to the left ankle (calcaneus and talus) in SK[8010], old adult male, Upton-on-Severn, Worcestershire. Note the secondary disuse atrophy of the left metatarsals. Right ankle normal.

(Ossafreelance)

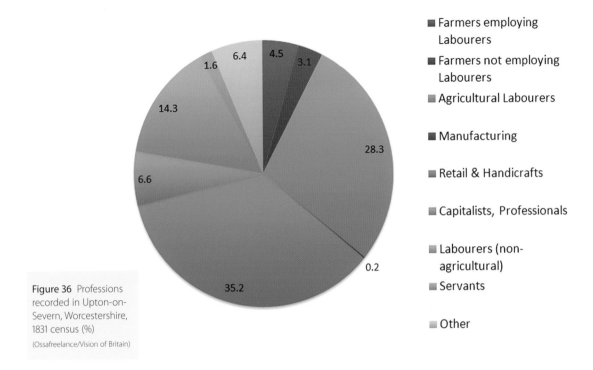

Legend:
- Farmers employing Labourers
- Farmers not employing Labourers
- Agricultural Labourers
- Manufacturing
- Retail & Handicrafts
- Capitalists, Professionals
- Labourers (non-agricultural)
- Servants
- Other

Pie chart values: 4.5, 3.1, 28.3, 0.2, 35.2, 6.6, 14.3, 1.6, 6.4

Figure 36 Professions recorded in Upton-on-Severn, Worcestershire, 1831 census (%)

(Ossafreelance/Vision of Britain)

individual had also suffered a fracture of the joint surfaces to the right ankle, which is likely to have occurred at the same time. This type of injury, known as a vertical compression fracture, is incurred through an individual falling from a considerable height and landing directly on their feet/heels. Severe comminuted fractures such as these (where the bone is shattered into several pieces) generally render the ankle irreparably damaged.

The contemporary census records for Upton-on-Severn tell us that the majority of males were employed in agriculture or in retail and handicraft (Fig. 36). A number of non-agricultural labourers were also present. In terms of socio-economic status, labourers and servants constituted 44.1% of the population while 38.4% were the 'middling sorts' (including small-scale farmers not employing labourers and masters, and skilled workers in the manufacturing and handicraft trades). Employers and professionals made up just 11.0% of the town's inhabitants. A substantial proportion of men in Upton-on-Severn then were manual labourers and farmers at considerable risk of occupational accidents such as falling from heights, leading to impact fractures like those seen in SK[8010].

Further evidence of the dangers of rural living was present in a skeletal assemblage from Stratford-upon-Avon. SK[906], a male over 50 years old, had five rib fractures

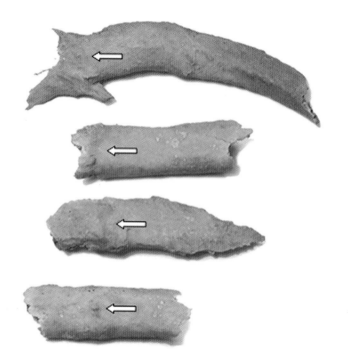

Figure 37 (left)
Multiple rib fractures,
(plural surface) healed,
SK[906], old adult
male, Industrial non-
metropolitan

(Ossafreelance)

Figure 38 (below)
Fractured right clavicle,
(posterior surface)
healed, SK[906], old adult
male, Industrial non-
metropolitan

(Ossafreelance)

(Fig. 37), a compression fracture of one upper/mid-thoracic vertebra, fracture of the right clavicle (collarbone: Fig. 38), fracture of the right ulna and radius (forearm) in the region of the wrist, fracture of the left distal fibula (lower leg) in the area of the ankle and an enthesophyte (bone spur) representing soft tissue trauma on the right femur (thighbone). It is highly likely that at least some of these injuries occurred at the same time and represent a high impact incident at some velocity, such as a fall from a height or involving a speeding carriage, for example.

High velocity injuries such as those seen in SK[906] often involved horse and cart road accidents. The increasing number of traffic accidents in Worcestershire

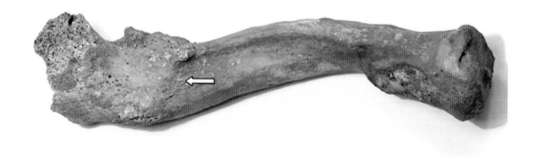

put a strain on the availability of hospital beds in the former Worcester Royal Infirmary which, in 1821, imposed charges of 7s 6d a week for board and lodging of patients to those 'who may be brought in from accidents, occasioned by improper or furious driving of public carriages, or vehicles of any description' in a bid to discourage dangerous driving. Some documented fatalities in rural locations were also contributed to by the poor state of privately maintained roads, leading to cartwheels hitting pot-holes, sometimes throwing passengers out of the cart onto the road at speed.

Coroner's records

Coroner's inquest records make for a gruesome and sobering read but provide first-hand witness accounts of accidents in the past (Fig. 39). The *Transcriptions of the Berrow's Index of Coroner's Cases* in Worcestershire and the West Midlands make reference to an inquest following the accidental death of an individual called Spicer on the 29 September 1814. The cause of death had only been entered as 'killed by cheese' but a detailed account of the incident was published in the Edinburgh Review of that year:

> September '17th – A most melancholy accident occurred on the turnpike road between Faringdon and Wantage, Berks. Mr. Spicer, a farmer, residing at Goosey, had loaded a waggon with cheese for Wantage, and his wife embraced the opportunity of riding in the waggon to that place: Having arrived opposite the farm, called Garlands, they were overtaken by some men, with a number of loose colts, returning from Lechlade fair; these, in passing, divided on each side of the waggon, and thereby frightened the horses which were drawing it; in endeavouring to stop them, the driver, John Combly, was beaten down, and both wheels passed over his loins – he expired in a few minutes afterwards. The horses set off at full gallop; the waggon was overturned and the cheese falling on Mrs Spicer, she was killed on the spot. The boy who led the fore horse had a narrow escape, having been knocked down by it, but he succeeded in rolling out of the way of the wheels before they passed.

A further horrific cart accident in one of our study areas at Shields, Tyneside was also detailed:

> September 13th 1814: On Monday se'ennight a melancholy accident happened on the Kenton waggon-way, near this town. A young woman named Margaret Dobson, in service at Shields, daughter of a waggonwoman at Coxlodge colliery, had leave to visit her parents and returning, she and another woman seated themselves on a board, behind her father's loaded coal waggon, to ride to

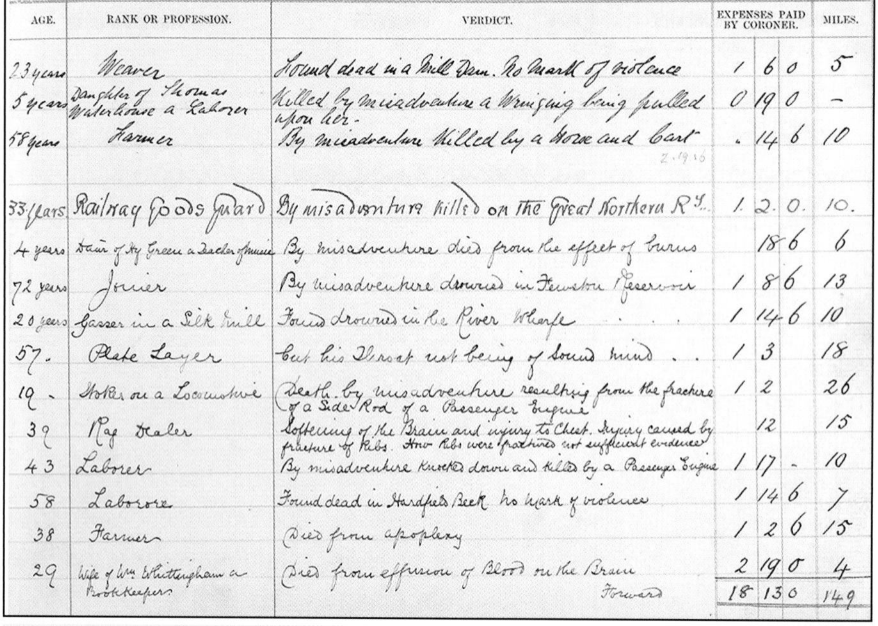

AGE.	RANK OR PROFESSION.	VERDICT.	EXPENSES PAID BY CORONER			MILES.
23 years	Weaver	Found dead in a Mill Dam. No mark of violence	1	6	0	5
5 years	Daughter of Thomas Waterhouse a Laborer	Killed by misadventure a Wringing being pulled upon her	0	19	0	-
58 years	Farmer	By misadventure killed by a Horse and Cart	.	14	6	10
		2.19.6				
33 years	Railway Goods Guard	By misadventure killed on the Great Northern R.Y.	1	2.0.		10.
4 years	Son of Joseph Green a Dealer of manure	By misadventure died from the effect of burns		18	6	6
72 years	Joiner	By misadventure drowned in Fewston Reservoir	1	8	6	13
20 years	Gasser in a Silk Mill	Found drowned in the River Wharfe	1	14	6	10
57.	Plate Layer	Cut his Throat not being of Sound mind	1	3		18
19 .	Stoker on a Locomotive	Death by misadventure resulting from the fracture of a Side Rod of a Passenger Engine	1	2		26
39	Rag Dealer	Softening of the Brain and injury to Chest. Injury caused by fracture of Ribs. How Ribs were fractured not sufficient evidence		12		15
43	Laborer	By misadventure knocked down and killed by a Passenger Engine	1	17	-	10
58	Laborer	Found dead in Hardfield Beck no mark of violence	1	14	6	7
38	Farmer	Died from apoplexy	1	2	6	15
29	Wife of Wm Whittingham a Bookkeeper	Died from effusion of Blood on the Brain	2	19	0	4
		Forward	18	13	6	149

Figure 39 Coroner's records for West Riding of Yorkshire, including Fewston, 1889

(public domain)

the Shields turnpike, over which the waggon-way passes. Near East Benton, a waggon which followed them at some distance ran amain, and they supposing it might be stopped before it reached them, did not move till it came too near, then M. Dobson, in endeavouring to escape, unfortunately slipped and fell with her neck across the cast metal rail, and the sharp metal wheels severed her head from her body. The other had her foot severely crushed.

Unfortunately, such accidental deaths were not one-off events. *The Transcriptions of the Berrow's Index of Coroner's Cases* reveals the unknown or sudden deaths of 24 individuals from Upton-upon-Severn between 1814 and 1833. Twelve of the individuals were identified as male and six female, with no biographical details for the remaining six. Unfortunately, the precise cause of death was not noted in most cases. However, four individuals had drowned accidentally and a further three men were identified as 'watermen'. One individual of unknown identity was also found dead in the river. In 1826 one unfortunate lady, Jane Williams, a brewer, was scalded in a skeel of hot wort (a tub of hot liquid extracted during the brewing process). In 1830, another woman had been administered a 'quantity of corrosive sublimate' in an attempt to induce an abortion by her husband, who was subsequently charged with her murder.

Sporting events, performing arts and entertainment were still largely unregulated in the early Industrial period, carrying not only a threat to the participants but also to large unruly crowds of onlookers. At Worcester in 1806, the Royal Infirmary treated two people for broken arms and tended a fatality as a result of a fairground accident, where people were thrown from 'a most ridiculous and dangerous piece of machinery called a "Merry-go-Round"'. Later, in 1824, doctors from the Infirmary were also required to attend an emergency on the Pitchcroft where thousands were attending a boxing match between the then renowned fighters Spring and Langan (Fig. 40). During the knock-out match,

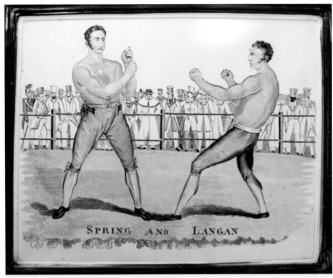

Figure 40 Commemorative ceramic plaque of Spring and Langan's famous match in Worcester, 1825

(public domain)

which lasted 80 rounds over a period of 2 hours and 32 minutes, one of the grandstands collapsed, the crowd falling 20 ft (6.1 m) below amid the broken timbers. The accident resulted in one fatality caused by a compound leg fracture and at least 30 people were taken to the Infirmary with serious fractures of the limbs or ribs. However, this did not stop the fight nor the appetite of the crowd, who eventually broke through the ring and encircled the fighting men who were then entrapped within a space of 8–10 ft (2.4–3 m) until the match was called to a halt.

Industrialising London: work rules

London became the largest city of the British Empire during the Industrial period, dominating the global stage in the political and economic spheres. Over the course of a century, the population rose from just under 1 million in 1801 to over 4.5 million in 1901. Despite the vast changes occurring in London, large mills and factories characteristic of the sprawling industrial northern cities did not loom large on the City's skyline. London's authority as the leading centre of trade was underpinned by its flourishing port on the Thames with its capacity to divert goods to and from the four corners of the globe. Commodities included silk, indigo, spices and also tea, which was worth £30 million pounds a year alone. In the 1840s, there were seven docks of immense scale that made up the City's port. London dock covered 90 acres (36 ha) of land. The Commercial, the Grand Surrey Canal and the East Country Dock on the South Bank covered almost 173 acres (70 ha) in total, 100 acres (nearly 40.5 ha) of that being water. New extensive docks at the Isle of Dogs, covering 54 acres (22 ha) in total, were constructed between 1800 and 1802 for the West India trading company, shortly followed by the East India Docks (Fig. 41) to the north-east. Although smaller, the East India docks could house 250 ships of up to a 1000 tons at any one time.

Many men worked not only at the dockyards and wharves throughout London but also, by this time, along the extensive network of subsidiary canals in the numerous trades attached to the waterways, such as rope making, ship building and in the transportation of raw and worked materials such as coal, ballast, bricks, timber and stone. Much of this work, prior to an Act of Parliament in 1848, was organised by publicans, who held workmen to ransom, awarding the day's work to those gangs of men who bought the most porter, rum or gin, or who lodged in their pubs. Payment to labourers still continued to be made in pubs even after 1848. Hard drinking was an integral and institutionalised part of a hard day's work, which only increased the risk of injury (Fig. 42). Labouring was primarily manual with some mechanical aids and accidents among the coal-whippers, ballast-getters, timber-lumpers and deal-porters were frequent. Slips and falls frequently resulted in broken legs and arms, often ill-set and sometimes hindering further physical capacity to work.

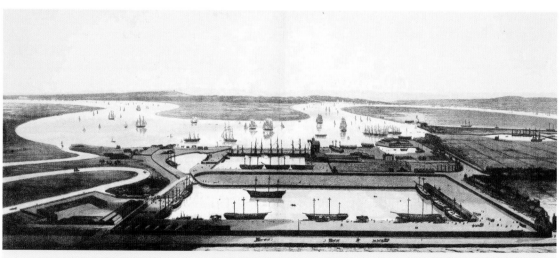

Figure 41 East India Dock, 1806
(Chronicles of Blackwall Yard by Robert Wigram and Henry Green, 1881, public domain)

The South Bank was the traditional location of industrial manufacturing activity, which had been banned from the City on account of its unpleasantness. Here, factories producing vinegar, dyes, soaps and tallow could be found alongside tanneries and timber yards (Fig. 43). The area was further industrialised after the building of Westminster Bridge in 1750 and Blackfriars Bridge in 1769 to include potteries, lime kilns and blacking factories. Bethnal Green and Spitalfields, meanwhile, became synonymous with cabinet making and textile production, which had had its roots in the medieval period but now rapidly became a mechanised trade employing most of the local population until its decline from the mid-19th century. Overall, by the 1840s, service and manufacturing industries provided most of the work in the City,

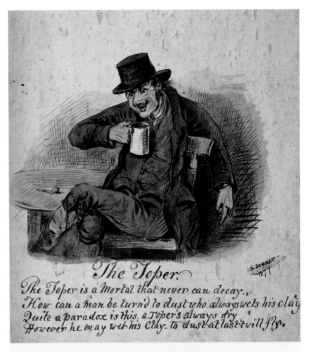

Figure 42 The Toper, or hardened drunkard, S. Jenner, 1877

(Wellcome Images)

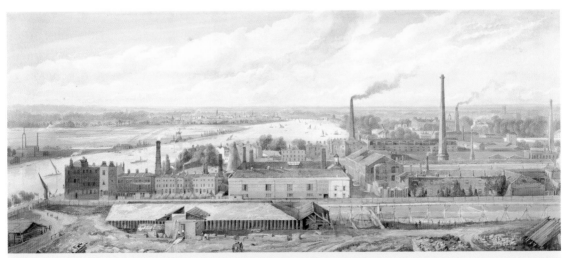

Figure 43 Panorama of the Thames from Millbank 19th century, 1845–1850

(© Museum of London)

the largest areas of employment being domestic servitude (168,000 workers), labouring (50,000), boot and shoemaking (28,000), tailors (23,500) and dressmakers (20,000).

Industrialisation led to the creation of job roles that were strictly defined and often gender specific. All the professions became hierarchical in their employment structure. As Henry Mayhew observed in the 1840s, 'society men' made up about 10% of a profession and had a very comfortable existence in well furnished, splendid houses, whereas the 'non-society men' were overworked and underpaid, 'so that a few week's sickness reduced them to absolute pauperism', living in 'squalor, misery, dirt, vice, ignorance and discontent' in areas like Spitalfields (Fig. 44) and Bethnal Green.

Men dominated occupations involving the operating of machinery, supervision, skilled labour and the heavy industry and construction fields. Low status women also worked in industry and manufacturing but were exploited for their cheap labour and very often worked from home on piece work to provide a supplementary income for their families in addition to running the household. Middle class women were also very often involved behind the scenes in businesses run by their husbands and undertook roles in retail, book keeping and correspondence. Retirement was rare. According to a survey of census records from 1891, 57% of people aged over 65 were employed, compared to only 10.1% of people in 2014, and this included 88% of all men.

To supplement the network of canals, inland transportation of much needed goods into the growing metropolis was facilitated by the London and Birmingham Railway's new intercity line, the first part of which opened in 1837 between Euston Station and Boxmoor (Hemel Hempstead, Hertfordshire). The construction of the line employed 20,000 men for 5 years. An Act of Parliament initially prevented locomotives from entering London beyond Camden Town, meaning that only fixed engines could be towed in by rope but this ceased in 1844. Inner city overground lines were introduced much later, from around the 1870s (Fig. 45). The London Underground's first line was opened in 1863, running gas-lit

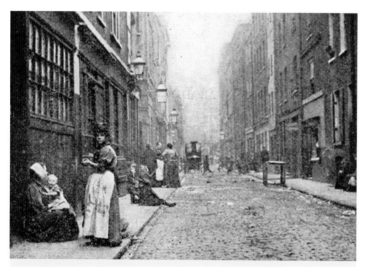

Figure 44 Dorset Street, Spitalfields, 1902
(public domain, CCO/1.0 Universal, https://commons.m.wikimedia.org/wiki/File:Dorset-street-1902.jpg#mw-jump-to-license)

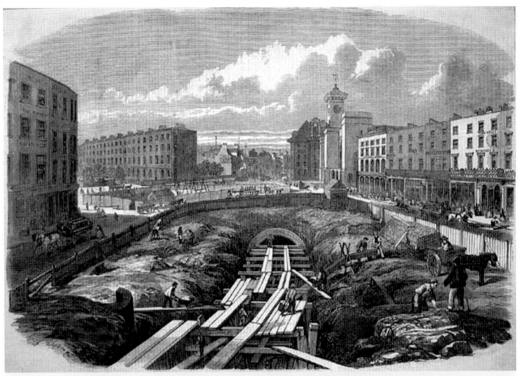

Figure 45 Constructing the Metropolitan Railway, near King's Cross Station, 1861
(Illustrated London News, cc-pd-mark, https://en.wikipedia.org/wiki/The_Illustrated_London_News, Public Domain)

wooden carriages hauled by steam locomotives between Paddington and Farringdon, and expanded over the same period of time as the overground lines (Fig. 46).

Between the 1830s and 1870s, the most common form of transportation was the horse-drawn carriage and the popular horse-drawn or steam-powered omnibuses (Fig. 47). Despite the *Locomotive Acts* or 'Red Flag Act' of 1836 limiting their speed to 3.2 km an hour in residential areas and enforcing every driver to have a rider 100 m in

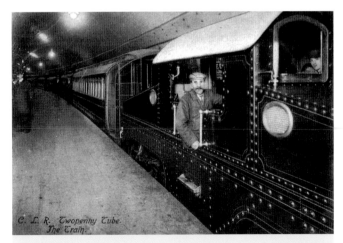

Figure 46 Central London Railway locomotive at Shepherd's Bush tube station, c. 1900–1903
(postcard, Unknown photographer, public domain, pd-uk, https://commons.wikimedia.org/wiki/File:Central_London_Railway_locomotive.png#filelinks)

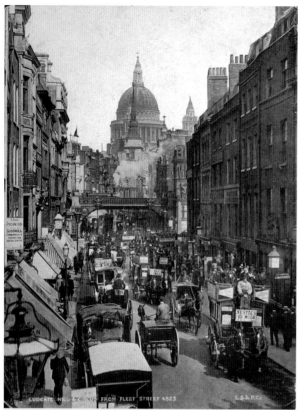

Figure 47 Postcard of Fleet Street, London, Ludgate Hill and Circus, 19th century

(© Museum of London)

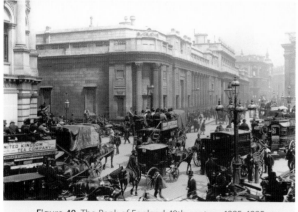

Figure 48 The Bank of England, 19th century, 1885–1895

(© Museum of London)

front waving a red flag to warn of the approaching vehicle, there were no further road safety regulations until the introduction of the motor car. As a result, the City's roads were a chaotic mix of steam-powered vehicles, horse-drawn carts, pedestrians and, from the 1880s, bicycles (Fig. 48). In 1890 there were 5728 street accidents resulting in 144 deaths.

Well-being became a fixation for the Victorians during the later Industrial period as part of a moral crusade to improve the lot of valuable employees. The regulation of sports was one aspect of this movement, aiming to instil moral values of fair play while simultaneously reducing injuries to their workers. Prize fighting, or bare knuckle boxing, was a sport rekindled in the early Industrial period, initially undertaken by skilled athletes who were sponsored by wealthy patrons. However, in the mid-18th century boxing was also enjoyed by 'persons of quality and distinction' who wore gloves to prevent 'black eyes, broken jaws and bloody noses', all deemed very off-putting at high society engagements (Fig. 49). The Boxing Academy, attended by such high status persons, was founded in 1714 in London. Fights between female pugilists were also surprisingly frequent, fought under the same rules as for men but often undertaken in alleyways outside pubs or in marketplaces, such as Billingsgate, between lower status females who struck blows, pulled hair and bit their opponents, sometimes while bare-chested. By the late Victorian period, prize fighting was discouraged as a morally repugnant activity, although boxing continued as a professional sport with the introduction of the Queensberry rules in 1867, ensuring that all fighters wore gloves.

Formal rules for football were first laid down in 1848 and Sheffield Football Club was the first team established in 1857, which played friendly matches against London and Nottingham. 'Football' was a bit of a misnomer at this stage as it was still a very hands-on game, whereby players were allowed to push and shove players off the ball and goalkeepers could be barged over the line if the football was in his hands. The first 11-a-side rules were created in 1862. A similar transformation occurred within the game of rugby, with the first rules being created in 1845, the Rugby Football Union eventually being formed in 1871 and a reduction in the number of players from 20 to 15 aside in 1877. In the later Victorian period, a rise in obesity among the middle classes was, for the social commentators, linked to moral turpitude and greed. This inspired some manufacturers to come up with exercise and stretching equipment for use in a home gym (Fig. 50), a trend that has continued ever since, though the clothing required at the time was much more formal!

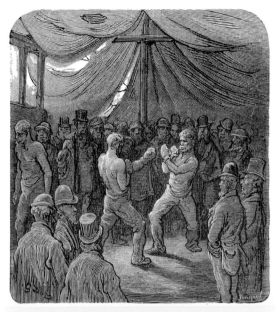

Figure 49 *The Noble Art* 1872, Gustave Dore
(© Museum of London)

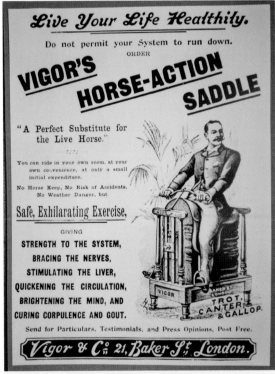

Figure 50 Advert for exercise horse
(public domain)

Broken bones: investigating trauma in the past

To investigate trauma in the past and any changes in fracture patterns over time, we examined the evidence for fractures of the cranium (skull), ribs, humerus (upper arm), radius/ulna (lower arm), hands, femur and tibia/fibula (leg bones) in Londoners and in people from outside the City, from both the Industrial and pre-Industrial periods (Fig. 51).

For crania, individuals were selected on the presence of at least half the cranial vault. For ribs, individuals were selected on the presence of at least one rib; for long bones, on the basis of having at least two-thirds of the selected element present, left or right side; for hands, on the presence of at least three phalanges (finger bones) over two anatomical rows of the fingers. Fractures to joints were not included. All individuals were of fair or good preservation. Average samples sizes were 1139 (Industrial London), 598 (pre-Industrial London), 533 (Industrial non-metropolitan)

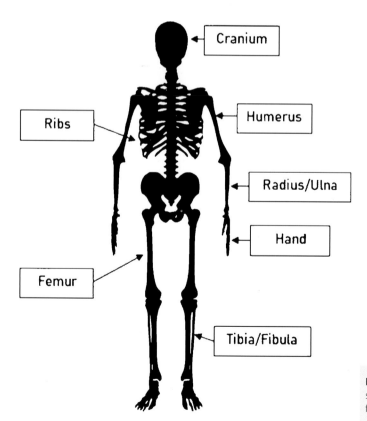

Figure 51 Identification of skeletal elements selected for trauma analysis

and 529 (pre-Industrial non-metropolitan) individuals. The samples consisted of males and females of either the young and middle age groups combined (20–49 years old) or the old adult age group (50+ years old) to assess any differences related to age and sex. For the London populations, we also examined the role of social status in fracture prevalence. In comparing fracture prevalence in past populations to modern populations, it must be remembered that in archaeological human skeletal remains we see evidence of healed trauma that has accumulated over an individual's life time. It is generally not possible to ascertain at what age an individual sustained an injury, unlike in modern populations where the age at which the fracture occurred is recorded. Our ability to identify age as a factor in fracture causation, therefore, can be limited.

Reference to clinical traumatology allows us to make inferences about the nature of fracture causation in the past. Most trauma seen in the skeleton is caused by either falls or blows. In the modern day context large robust bones in healthy individuals, such as the femur, are frequently broken in high energy accidents like car and motorbike collisions due to the major force required to fracture such a robust bone (Table 2). Less robust bones can be fractured more easily from lower energy impacts. The elderly are more vulnerable to fractures because of the ageing process leading to less dense bone structure and in some cases, osteoporosis. Additionally, smoking has been identified as not only an increased risk factor of bone fracture but also contributing towards slower healing.

Table 2 Fracture Aetiology

Skeletal element	Force required	Aetiology
Femur	High energy impact	Road accident, fall from height, gunshot
Tibia (severe fracture)	High energy impact	Road accident, fall from height
Tibia (simple)	Low energy impact	Athletic injuries, falls
Skull	High energy impact	Falls, traffic accidents, sports injuries, assaults
Humerus	Low energy impact	Fall onto outstretched arm or direct impact on arm
Radius/Ulna	Low energy impact	Fall onto outstretched arm or direct impact on arm
Ribs	Low energy impact	Blunt force trauma following falls, non-accidental injury, severe coughing, athletic activities
Hands	Low energy impact	Falls, crush or twisting injuries, direct contact often occurring in sports

The skeletal evidence: trauma in London compared to outside the city

In all groups, the most commonly affected anatomical area was the ribs followed by either hand or lower arm. The least affected elements in the majority of groups were the humerus and femur/hip (Table 3). The low level of femoral fractures (Figs 52 and 53) suggests that high impact accidents were relatively uncommon in all our past populations, even during the Industrial period. Most common was blunt force trauma to the chest, trauma to the hands (Figs 54 and 55) and low impact falls onto outstretched arms. Skull fractures and low impact falls involving the lower leg were consistently present in all our groups but were of a relatively low frequency.

During the pre-Industrial period, the overall rates of fractures outside of the City were significantly higher than those in London. However, evidence for trauma significantly increased over time in London. Conversely, in areas outside London, rates of trauma decreased over time. By the Industrial period, there was no significant difference between rates of trauma in London and those areas outside of the City (Fig. 56).

Within industrial London, the higher status groups at Chelsea, Hackney and from St Bride's crypt had modest rates of rib fractures, ranging from 7.1% to 9.8%. The highest rates of rib fractures were amongst the low status groups from the densely occupied Lower St Bride's in central London (20.5%) and Bethnal Green (16.1%). However, the lowest rate of rib fractures was found at Bow (5.5%). Despite its low social status, Bow was an area that, unlike the City and Bethnal Green, only became urbanised from around 1850 and had an economic history generally associated only with light industry and markets until this date. By 1853, the Baptists' burial ground had closed so the skeletal assemblage pre-dates the more intense industrialisation of the area. Outside of London in the Industrial period, rib fractures were lower in the

Table 3 Elements in order of most frequent to least frequently affected in each group

Industrial London	%	Pre-Industrial London	%	Industrial non-metropolitan	%	Pre-Industrial non-metropolitan	%
Ribs	12.8	Ribs	3.1	Ribs	8.6	Ribs	10.7
Hand	6.0	Radius/Ulna	3.0	Hand	5.9	Radius/Ulna	6.4
Radius/Ulna	2.5	Hand	1.7	Radius/Ulna	3.7	Hand	5.3
Tibia/Fibula	2.4	Tibia/Fibula	1.7	Tibia/Fibula	3.2	Tibia/Fibula	3.6
Skull	2.1	Skull	1.6	Femur	0.9	Skull	2.9
Humerus	1.2	Femur	0.5	Skull	0.8	Femur	0.5
Femur	1.0	Humerus	0.0	Humerus	0.5	Humerus	0.4

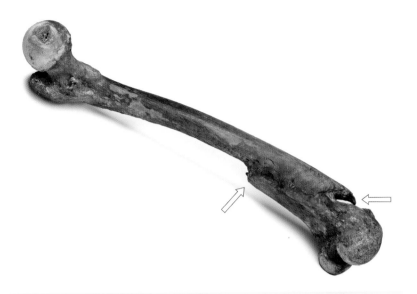

Figure 52 Healed fracture of left femur, middle adult male from Industrial London (PGV10 2588)

(© Museum of London)

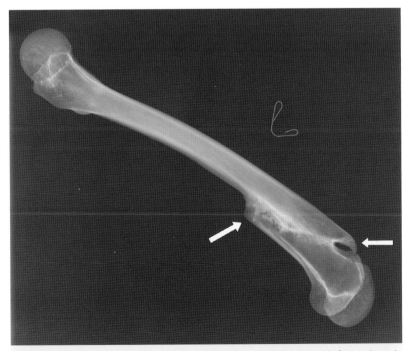

Figure 53 Digital radiograph of healed fractured left femur, middle adult male from Industrial London (PGV10 2588)

(© Museum of London)

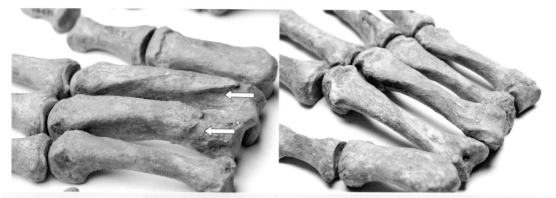

Figure 54 Healed fractures of the left hand in the 2nd and 3rd metacarpal (arrowed), the right hand no fractures of the metacarpals, middle adult female, pre-Industrial London (SRP98 6775)

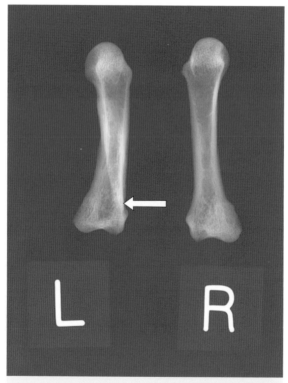

Figure 55 Digital radiograph of left and right 2nd metacarpal (hand bones) with the left 2nd metacarpal showing a healed fracture of the shaft, middle adult female, pre-Industrial London (SRP98 6775)

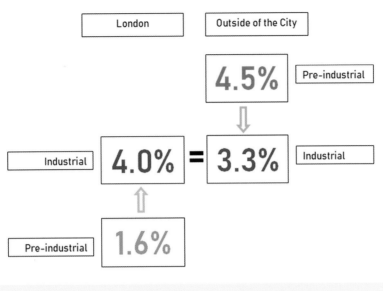

Figure 56 Rates of fractures over time in London and outside of the City

larger towns at North Shields and at Swinton (average 4.2%) compared to towns and villages in more rural locations, such as Upton-on-Severn, Fewston and Stratford-upon-Avon (average 11.9%), where subsistence relied heavily on agricultural economies.

Trauma in males
- Prior to industrialisation, younger males living outside London were more at risk of trauma than those living in London. Total rates of fractures (3.9%) and rib fracture rates (10.3%) were much higher outside the City than in it (1.7% and 3.3% respectively).
- By the Industrial period in London, rates of rib (11.1%) and hand fractures (6.8%) had risen in younger males compared to the pre-Industrial period (3.3% and 2.2% respectively). Conversely, there was no increased risk of trauma over time for younger males outside the City. The importance of occupation and lifestyle was also evident in industrial London, where younger males of low social status experienced a higher risk of hand fractures (9.4%) than higher status males (1.1%).
- A similar pattern was seen in old aged males, with higher rates of rib fractures (24.8%) and total fractures (9.3%) in males from outside the City during the pre-Industrial period than in London (8.8% and 2.8% respectively) but with the same fractures increasing in number over time in the City in the Industrial period (23.5% and 7.6% respectively) and, in particular, for low status males (31.4% and 9% respectively). Outside of the City, rates of fractures present in old age males did not change significantly over time.

Overall, while the risk of trauma in the City grew over time, in small towns and villages in more rural areas industrialisation had a minimal impact on the overall exposure of younger males to trauma. This was due to the continuation of the pre-existing significant risk from rural lifestyles and occupations. Overall, the risk of trauma during the Industrial period was the same for males both within and outside of the City (Fig. 57).

Trauma in females
- Amongst younger females, those from the pre-Industrial populations outside the City had the highest overall rate of fractures (2.7%). Rates of fractures to the radius/ulna (6.8%) were higher in the pre-Industrial younger females from outside of London than either their contemporaries in London (3.3%) or later industrial populations located either in the City (0.6%) or outside it (1.1%).

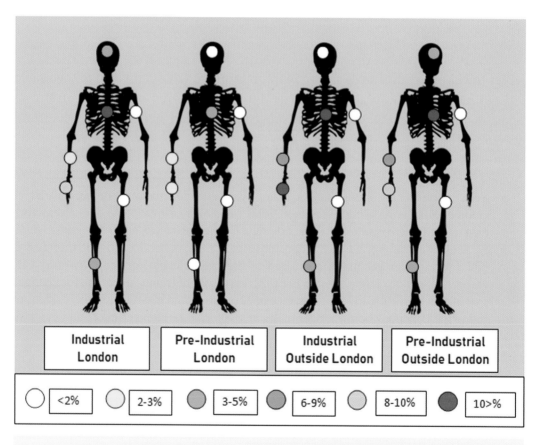

Figure 57 Comparative fracture rates, males, all age groups

- The highest rate of rib fractures was in younger females from Industrial London (6.3%), with a significant increase in rates over time from the pre-Industrial period (1.7%). However, unlike their male counterparts, this rise in trauma in younger females in the City over time was not related to social status.

In conclusion, younger females living outside the City in the pre-Industrial period were at the highest risk of trauma, though this decreased over time. Within London, rates of trauma in younger females involving some skeletal elements increased over time, though overall rates remained relatively constant (Fig. 58).

In the old aged female group, few fractures were reported in either the Industrial period populations from outside the City or from the pre-Industrial population within the City. To a certain extent, this may reflect the smaller sample size of females in the older age group who were under-represented in some populations compared to

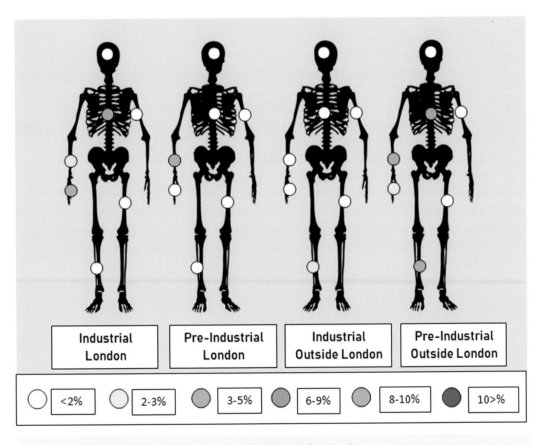

Figure 58 Comparative fracture rates, females, all age groups

male old aged adults. The risk of trauma in old age females, however, largely followed the same patterns as their male counterparts, though not always.

- In the pre-Industrial period, no significant differences in fracture rates were found between the old age female Londoners and those outside the City.
- In Industrial London, the overall rate of trauma in old aged females (3.9%) was higher than in their contemporaries outside the City (1.3%), particularly with regard to rib fractures (10.6% v 1.4% only).
- There was a significantly higher level of trauma in the lower status old aged females in Industrial London, who experienced significantly higher rates of hand fractures (9.8%) than their high status counterparts (0%).

The combined roles of age, sex and status
- Before the industrialisation of the City, males and females at any age were equally at risk of trauma in London (1.9% v 1.2%).
- During the Industrial period in London, the rate of trauma for males became more than double the rate of trauma for females (5.5% v 2.5%).
- Outside the City, the prevalence of trauma in males compared to females was consistently higher over time.
- In Industrial London, age became a significant factor in risk of trauma. Higher rates of rib fractures and overall skeletal trauma were present in older males compared to younger males.
- This was a pattern repeated outside of the City, where rates of rib, hand and total number of fractures were higher in old age males than in younger males in the Industrial period.
- Significantly more trauma was also seen in old age females compared to younger females in the Industrial period but only in London. Outside the city, this was not the case and similar levels of trauma were seen in younger and old age females.
- The increasing risk of trauma with age for females in London varied according to social status. There were a significantly higher number of fractures in low status females of old age compared to their younger counterparts. This was not evident in high status females.
- This pattern was also seen in males. Low status old aged adult males in the City had significantly more fractures than lower status younger males, a pattern that was not reflected in their high status contemporaries.

Overall, the industrialisation of London led to a significant increase in fractures and key factors in this increase were social status and age. Both males and females of low status in London were at much higher risk of experiencing trauma by old age. Being of higher status during the Industrial period reduced the risk of fractures over the lifetime of both males and females in London. Outside of the City, although age was a factor in males and females experiencing increased trauma, industrialisation was not. In fact, industrialisation led to a decrease in trauma in females.

Interpersonal violence

Sharp force trauma in the skeleton, most frequently seen on the skull consisting of blade wounds and cuts, is the clearest evidence we have for violent attacks in the past. Blunt force trauma is commonly associated with violent assaults but, unfortunately, it is rarely possible for osteoarchaeologists to differentiate between blunt force trauma caused by accidental falls or by intentional blows. It is also very rare to see evidence for sharp force trauma to the chest as it usually affects soft tissues only.

Overall, rates of cranial trauma, including both sharp force and blunt force, were fairly consistent across the Industrial and pre-Industrial populations, both in and outside the City. One exception was a significant fall in overall cranial trauma seen outside London over time, from 2.9% to 0.8%, with the highest rate of cranial trauma being recorded in the pre-Industrial non-metropolitan population. There was no significant difference in sharp force trauma prevalence in any of the populations and there was no influence of social status on either total crania trauma, blunt force trauma or sharp-force only cranial trauma.

Nasal fractures (Fig. 59) are very often associated with interpersonal violence and athletic injuries but can also less commonly occur as the result of falls or accidents. As with cranial trauma, there was no significant difference in rates of nasal trauma between social groups in London. Low status males did have significantly more nasal fractures than females (7.0% v 0.9%), however, whereas there was no significant difference between males and females (3.7% v 1.4%) in high status groups.

This may reflect a tendency for low status males to have become embroiled in interpersonal violence, as is the trend today, though not to the extent that rates of nasal fractures were significantly more frequent than in high status males, whose refined cultural sporting hobbies still led them to violent encounters on occasion. Amongst labourers, Henry Mayhew identified institutionalised alcohol consumption as a major factor in violent activity. He was informed by one wife of her husband that, 'He often comes home and ill-uses me ... he beats me with his fists, he strikes me in the face, he has kicked me. When he was sober he was a good kind husband.'

Numbers of violent deaths amongst young adults were double that of old aged individuals between 1851 and 1860 according to data from the General Registrar's records. In our sample, 5.9% of deaths were related to violence in young adults, compared to 5.2% in middle aged adults and 2.9% of old adults (Fig. 60). Hotspots for violent deaths in all age groups were notably those with high levels of population density and economic deprivation, both inside and outside London. High status Chelsea had the lowest level of violent deaths (2.0%) whereas Spitalfields had the highest level (8.9%). Whereas pre-urbanisation, low levels of skeletal trauma were seen in Bow, after

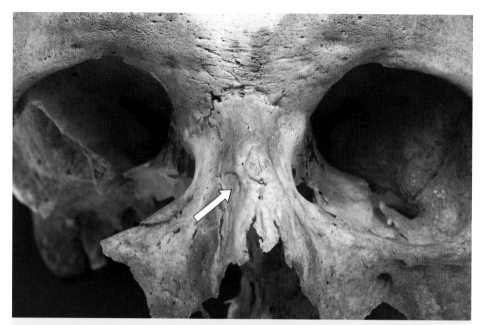

Figure 59 Healed nasal fracture, middle adult male from Industrial London (FAO90 1797)

(© Museum of London)

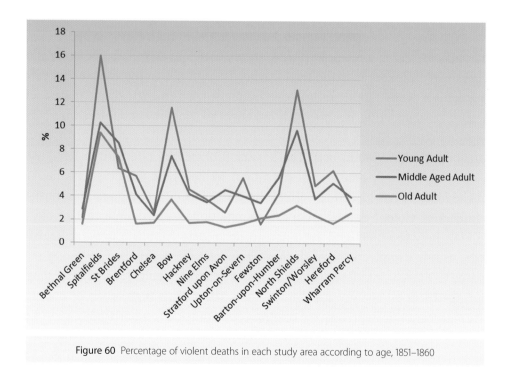

Figure 60 Percentage of violent deaths in each study area according to age, 1851–1860

urbanisation had started the area experienced high levels of violent deaths compared to other areas in the City. Outside London, the highest level was in North Shields (7.1%) compared to Stratford-upon-Avon, which had the lowest level (2.2%).

The history of health and safety and road safety

By the beginning of the 19th century, the consequences of the rapid rate of industrialisation and the dangers of the use of powered technology in the work-place were brought to the attention of Parliament, who acted not only to limit the harsh conditions found in factories and mills but also to enhance the education of apprentices. The first Act of Parliament introduced to protect the welfare of workers was the *Factory Act* 1802, which was passed with almost no opposition. Focused largely on eliminating the misuse of children in textile mills, the Act legislated for improved cleanliness and ventilation in the work-place and to restrict working hours for some pauper apprentices to 12 hours a day. Magistrates were charged with inspecting the factories and the responsibility of also ensuring that apprentices received basic education in reading, writing, arithmetic and religion.

However, due to the evasion of this new legislature, further Acts were introduced, culminating in the 1833 *Factories Act.* This new Act was broader in scope and restricted working days to 10 hours for all children and made it illegal to employ any child under the age of 9 years old. Most importantly, in tandem, the HM Factory Inspectorate was formed, comprising four independent inspectors who had the powers to enter mills, question workers and to formulate new regulations and laws to ensure the enforcement of this new Act. In 1837, the first case came to court that established an obligation of an employer towards the welfare of an employee whereby if breached and an injury had occurred, the employee could pursue the employer legally. The *Coal Mines Act* of 1842 prevented all women and children working underground. Meanwhile, the Inspectorate started to have a positive effect and by 1868 there were 35 inspectors and furthermore, between 1860 and 1871, legislation evolved to encompass all work-places within its provision, so that Acts in the workplace by 1900 covered coal mines, factories, mills, quarries, threshing and chaff cutting machinery. Employers responsibilities towards their employees was extended by the *Employers Liability Act* in 1880 to protect workers from accidents caused by negligent managers, superintendents and foremen and specifically within the railway companies, for accidents caused by signalmen, drivers and pointsmen. Safety, health and welfare in agriculture were only legislated for in 1956. The most comprehensive set of laws for the general workplace finally arrived in the form of the *Health and Safety at Work Act* 1974; leading to the creation of the Health and Safety Commission and Health and Safety Executive, which still operates today. The introduction of the *Health and Safety at Work Act* led to a staggering fall in the number of fatal injuries by 73% between 1974 and 2007, with non-fatal injuries also falling by 70%.

No. 2. "I am going to TURN to my RIGHT."

(This signal may be used in any circumstances when it may be necessary to convey the warning "It is DANGEROUS to OVERTAKE me on my RIGHT").

Extend the right arm and hand, <u>with the palm turned to the front,</u> and hold them *rigid* in a horizontal position straight out from the off side of the vehicle.

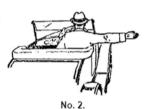

No. 2.

No. 3." You may OVERTAKE me on my RIGHT."

(This signal should only be given when it is safe for the overtaking vehicle to pass. **The overtaking driver is not absolved thereby from the duty of satisfying himself that he can overtake with safety.**)

Extend the right arm and hand <u>below</u> the level of the shoulder and move them backwards and forwards.

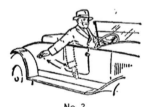

No. 3.

The drivers of HORSE-DRAWN vehicles should preferably use the three foregoing signals, giving them where possible by hand alone, and in any case keeping the whip (if any) clear of other traffic.

Alternatively, the following signals may be used :—

No. 4. "I am going to STOP."

Raise the whip vertically with the arm extended above the right shoulder.

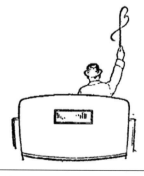

Figure 61 Illustrations from the Highway Code, introduced in 1931 (Ministry of Transport)

Outside of the workplace, by 1916, the danger of road traffic and driving in the City had become of such concern that the London 'Safety First' Council was elected to tackle the 'alarming increase in traffic accidents'. Safe driving competitions for professional drivers employed in Greater London were set up in 1917 and the notion was raised that all drivers should be licensed and their age restricted. The pedestrian rule was amended so that pedestrians faced oncoming traffic, leading to a dramatic reduction of pedestrian fatalities by 70% in the first 12 months. In 1917, 660 people were killed on the streets of London as the result of accidents. Although this decreased by 8% in the following year, in 1919, a railway strike led a 10% increase in road accidents. The railways themselves were still relatively dangerous and in 1921, 991 people died in railway accidents.

Motor vehicles, however, were by far the most common mode of transport involved in traffic accidents, numbers of which increased year upon year. In 1926, 4886 people were killed on the roads which rose dramatically to 9169 deaths in 1941. The introduction of several measures (Fig. 61), such as speed limits, enforcement technologies, motorways, the enforced used of seat belts and restrictions on alcohol consumption before driving, have ensured a substantial reduction in the number of road fatalities across the country, from a peak of 7985 in 1966 to 1792 in 2016.

Accidents and violence today

The pattern of fractures found in our archaeological populations is in contrast with modern populations in the UK where, although hand and lower arm fractures are still the most common form of skeletal trauma, femur/hip and humerus fractures are relatively more frequent than in our past populations. This indicates that there is a higher proportion of high energy impact trauma today than in the past, most likely due to motor vehicle accidents at speed. Rib and skull fractures are the least commonly reported type of fracture in modern populations. Rib fractures may be under-reported, however because some people do not seek medical treatment.

Injuries are reported as the age-standardised rate of mortality from injuries in persons less than 75 years of age per 100,000 from 2014–2016. The highest rate of mortality is recorded in Fewston (15.1), followed by Barton-upon-Humber (14.2) (Fig. 62), while the lowest rates are at Chelsea (9.1) and Brentford, outer London (8.5) (Fig. 63).

This suggests a reversal of the trend towards increased trauma levels in the City as a result of industrialisation. Today, as in the pre-Industrial past, rates of injuries are

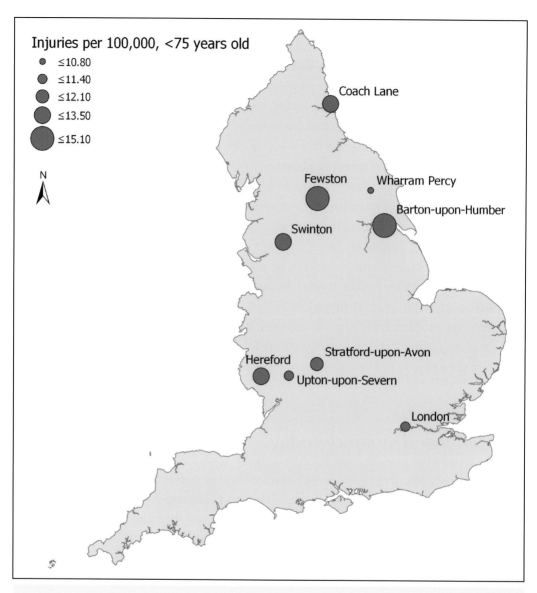

Figure 62 National sites showing injuries per 100,000 population for <75 years olds (Public Health England, 2014–2016)

once again higher outside of the City in more rural settings. However, a more complex picture emerges when looking at the statistics for those killed or seriously injured on the roads. Overall, more road traffic accident black spots occur in rural locations (Fig. 64). Excluding Central London, rates of road injuries and deaths are still lower in the City than our study areas outside of London (average of 29.6 compared to 42.6). However, Central London itself has one of the highest rates overall at 64.3 per

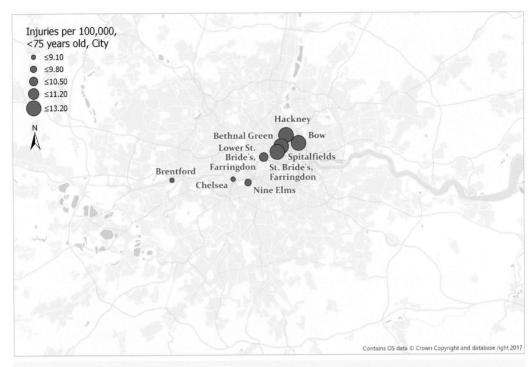

Figure 63 London sites showing injuries per 100,000 population for <75 years olds (Public Health England, 2014–2016)

100,000 (Fig. 65). The national average is 38.5 per 100,000. Even though Central London is one of the least densely inhabited areas of the City, the sheer volume of people and traffic travelling through the City centre using multiple forms of transport is still creating high levels of road fatalities (Fig. 66). Conversely, rates of mortality from non-road related injuries are highest in the lower status east end areas of Hackney (13) and Tower Hamlets (13), outside of Central London (10.5) and high status areas such as Chelsea (9.1).

Thanks to modern health and safety regulations, deaths within the work-place in 2017–8 in Great Britain were very low, numbering a total of 144 workers or 0.45 deaths per 100,000 workers, a reduction from around 2.0–2.5 deaths per 100,00 in the 1980s. Based on an absolute count of fatalities alone, most deaths occurred in the construction industry (38), closely followed by agriculture (29) and manufacturing (15). However, when taking into account the number of workers in each industry, the waste industry and agriculture have considerably higher relative rates of fatalities, with rates of injury being 18 and 16 times those of the average. There is actually comparatively less risk in the construction industry, where the rate is only four times the average rate. The most common cause of death was falling from a

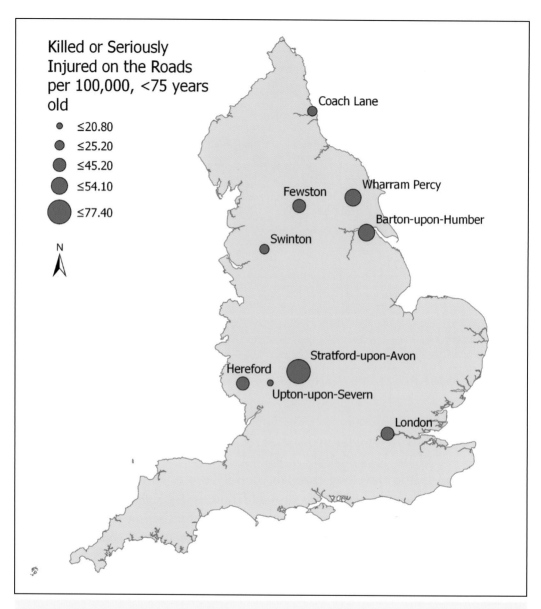

Killed or Seriously Injured on the Roads per 100,000, <75 years old

- ● ≤20.80
- ● ≤25.20
- ● ≤45.20
- ● ≤54.10
- ● ≤77.40

N

Coach Lane

Fewston

Wharram Percy

Barton-upon-Humber

Swinton

Stratford-upon-Avon

Hereford

Upton-upon-Severn

London

Figure 64 National statistics for killed or seriously injured on the roads per 100,000 population, <75 years old (Public Health England, 2014–2016)

height (35), followed by being struck by a moving vehicle (26) or object (23). Other causes were being trapped (something collapsing or overturning) (16), contact with moving machinery (13), injured by an animal (9), slips, trips or falls on the same level (4), drowning (3), contact with electricity (3) and exposure to fire (3). Almost all worker fatalities occurred in males (96%) and nearly 40% of these were over 60

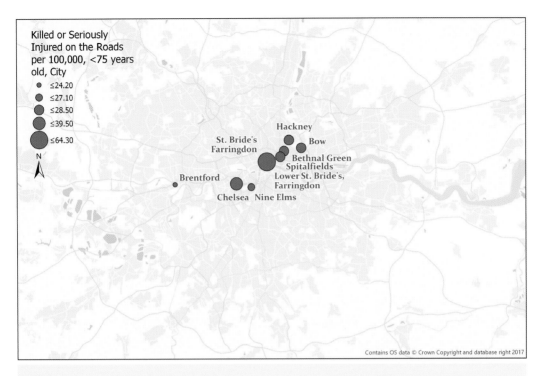

Killed or Seriously Injured on the Roads per 100,000, <75 years old, City

- ● ≤24.20
- ● ≤27.10
- ● ≤28.50
- ● ≤39.50
- ● ≤64.30

N

Hackney
St. Bride's Farringdon
Bow
Bethnal Green
Spitalfields
Brentford
Lower St. Bride's, Farringdon
Chelsea   Nine Elms

Contains OS data © Crown Copyright and database right 2017

Figure 65 London statistics for killed or seriously injured on the roads per 100,000 population, <75 years old (Public Health England, 2014–2016)

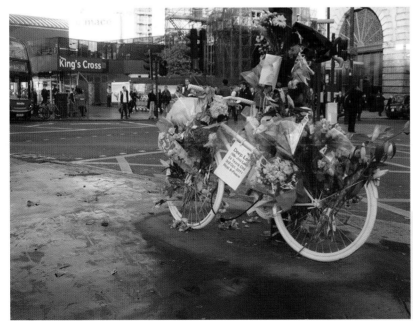

Figure 66 Ghost bike, a tribute to a road traffic accident fatality in the city

(cc-by-sa/2.0 © Stephen McKay, https://www.geograph.org.uk/photo/2699228)

years old, despite only making up approximately 10% of the workforce. No significant differences in rates of worker mortality occur between different regions or countries within Great Britain. Work-related deaths involving members of the public totalled 100 in 2017–8, with 51 of these occurring on railways and 16 in the health and social work sector.

Today, knife crime in the capital is tragically on the rise, with the media recently highlighting the shocking 22% rise of offences involving knives in 2017 in England and Wales. In past populations, the limited evidence from skeletal remains suggests that sharp force trauma, to the head at least, occurred at a relatively low rate that was fairly consistent on a national level. In comparison based on police recorded offences data for 2016/2017, knife crime involving attempted murder, homicide, actual bodily harm and grievous bodily harm was far higher in London than in other areas (Table 4).

The debate regarding the explanation for the rise in knife crime, which most often involves young males, has highlighted the role social media might have in providing a means of promoting acts of revenge violence. However, youth workers emphasise that social media can also empower young people and they stress that issues surrounding violent behaviours often have roots in economic deprivation, a lack of motivation and of future aspirations. Others point to cuts in police funding and anger against their stop and search policies (Fig. 67).

Levels of violent behaviour at sporting events are still a concern, as is crowd safety and culpability following the mass fatalities occurring at the Hillsborough stadium football disaster in 1989 in which 96 people died and 766 were injured. Thankfully, however, fatalities as a result of sporting injuries are very rare due to the regulated

Table 4 Knife crime incidents in 2016/7 involving attempted murder, homicide, actual bodily harm and grievous bodily harm (population figures rounded to hundreds)

Region	No. of reports	Population	per 100,000
Metropolitan London	5511	8778500	62.8
City of London	9	9400	95.7
Northumbria	282	1444800	19.5
North Yorkshire	171	813200	21.0
Humberside	248	927900	26.7
West Mercia	301	1258700	23.9
Warwickshire	135	556800	24.2
Greater Manchester	772	2782100	27.7

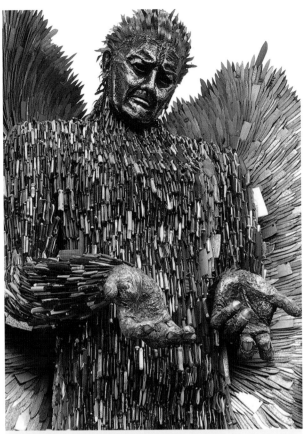

Figure 67 The Knife Angel sculpture, national monument against violence and aggression, Hull

(Dom Fellowes, cc-by/2.0, https://www.flickr.com/photos/domfell/40109423003)

nature of modern-day sports, though exact data on sporting injuries in the UK is lacking. Most preventative measures have focused on reducing the risk of head injuries through either restricted body contact or the introduction of protective head gear. One area still being investigated is the putative link between chronic traumatic encephalopathy or CTE (which can eventually lead to dementia) and repetitive low level head trauma, such as might be sustained in boxing or by heading a football. Although a link is suspected, no conclusive evidence has yet been found.

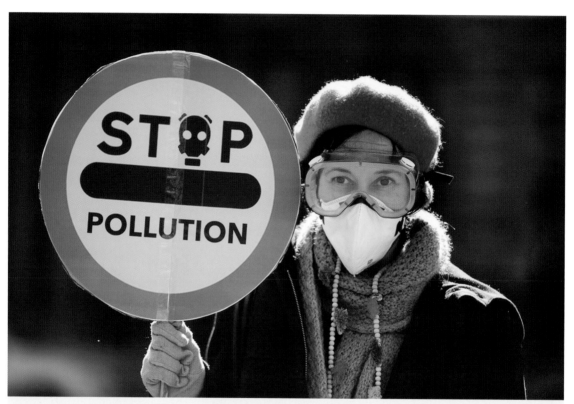

Figure 68 Environmental Protester

(Ian MacNicol / Friends of the Earth Scotland)

2

The air we breathe

The direct impact of the wider physical environment on our health is never more evident than in the quality of the air we breathe (Fig. 69). Today, 'Smog day' hopes to raise awareness of the estimated 18,000 people around the world who die prematurely every day as a result of air pollution. We all need clean air to breathe but, through-

out history, achieving the balance between human endeavour and human health has proved to be a challenge. In the UK this is epitomised by the Industrial period. Industrialisation brought about severe impacts on air quality throughout the Victorian period, exemplified frequently in human skeletal remains by the presence of rickets in children, brought about by an underexposure to vitamin D caused by smog blocking out the sunlight. Coal burning remained popular until at least the mid-20th century, when more than 200 million tonnes of coal were being used annually in England and Wales. Areas where rates of coal burning was high, especially

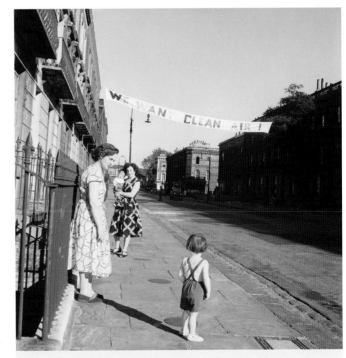

Figure 69 'We Want Clean Air' protest banner at Paddington, 1956
(© Henry Grant Collection/Museum of London)

for domestic use, have been shown to have significant increases in risk of mortality from not only respiratory conditions such as chronic obstructive pulmonary disease, pneumonia and tuberculosis but also epithelial cancers, particularly those of the respiratory tract and the upper gastrointestinal cancers. New medical research has now also identified air pollution as a trigger for diabetes by demonstrating that pollutants entering the bloodstream interact with organs, including liver tissue, to promote a domino effect of cellular reactions that leads to glucose intolerance. Research published in the *Lancet Planetary Health* in 2018 indicates a consistent association between increased $PM_{2.5}$ (fine particulate matter) and diabetes, as well all cause mortality.

Major concerns have been raised about carbon dioxide and sulphur dioxide churned out by vehicles, power plants and factories burning fossil fuels such as coal, and this alarm about the effects of polluted air on local living environments in fact is nothing new.

More recently, however, other 'greenhouse gases' such as methane and chlorofluorocarbons (CFCs) have also come into question in the wake of global climatic changes. We are all now very aware of the push towards us reducing our carbon footprints but what exactly is air pollution, where does it come from and how has it affected our health over time?

Air at work and home

Air pollution can take many forms. Not only can these consist of foreign particles from the wider environment but also those from our own lifestyle habits, such as tobacco smoking (Fig. 70), burning coal or wood within the home, or from our working environments, like inhaling occupational dust from manufacturing. These too can have serious consequences. In 2015, smoking was recorded as contributing

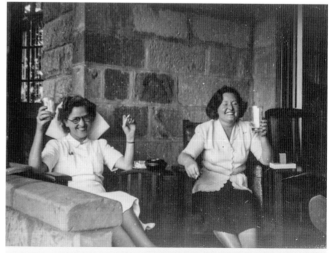

Figure 70 Two nurses smoking on a break, undated

towards approximately 105,000 deaths in the UK (that's 19% of all deaths of all causes) even though there has been a continual gradual decline in smoking since the 1940s. Second-hand smoke consumed through passive smoking is estimated to contribute to 11,000 deaths in the UK. In 2012, after the *Health Act* 2006 ensuring smoke free workplaces, 80% of these deaths were due to inhalation of second-hand smoke in the home compared to 20% in the workplace. Inhalation of other manufacturing related irritants were commonly referred to during the early years of medicine. Practitioners during the Victorian period noted high prevalence rates of 'inflammation of the lungs' caused by ceramic dust in towns producing pottery such as Stafford and Worcester, leading to the recognition of 'occupational diseases'. A more recent concern of the same issue was asbestos, banned in 1999 in the UK due to its fatal effects.

Airborne diseases

We may also come into contact with airborne pathogens by cramming ourselves into crowded spaces, such as busy shops, offices and commuter trains. This can lead to increased exposure to pathogens exhaled into the air by infected people and thereby causing rising levels of lung inflammation, either directly or by exacerbating pre-existing illnesses. Prior to the discovery of antibiotics and the implementation of

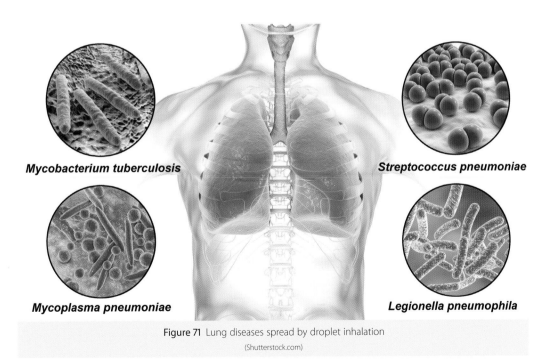

Mycobacterium tuberculosis

Streptococcus pneumoniae

Mycoplasma pneumoniae

Legionella pneumophila

Figure 71 Lung diseases spread by droplet inhalation
(Shutterstock.com)

vaccination schemes, some of these diseases were not only chronic but also could be fatal for large numbers of people. This is particularly true of respiratory or pulmonary tuberculosis, a disease which still exists today in the UK but in much reduced numbers of individuals (6520 cases in 2014).

It is spread by infected airborne droplet inhalation and is very much seen as a disease of poverty and overcrowding. In the past, this was a leading killer of young and middle aged adults, accounting for 30–40% of all deaths in this age group between 1851 and 1860. Other 'lung' diseases were also a high contributor to mortality rates amongst old age adults in the same period, though this classification is a general categorisation of a range of numerous diseases of the lung, including diseases of the respiratory system, influenza, pneumonia and bronchitis (Fig. 71).

Pre-Industrial London: the burning question

Air quality in London is currently reputed to be amongst the worst globally; a far cry from the description of the City in *c.* 1173 by William Fitz Stephen as 'happy in the healthiness of its air'. It has thought to have been on the decline since the 13th century when air pollution was linked not only to coal burning but also to the lime burning industry in the City. Seacole (sea coal) was brought to London from Newcastle from the 13th century originally as ballast, shortly after which it was burnt primarily as part of lime production but was also used by blacksmiths. Subsequently, its impressive heat production qualities lead to its rapid adoption in further industries in the City, such as brewing. However, the obnoxious smell accompanying the burning was the source of numerous complaints by high status occupants and visitors to London. Thus, the use of coal in domestic settings in England was not popular and was certainly not entertained in the culinary sphere, the preference being for using wood as fuel.

Initially, there was a fear that the burning of seacoles, so evident by the pungent smell emitted, would have adverse effects on health. Commissions were set up in 1285 and 1288 to investigate alternative sources of heat production, and in 1307 a proclamation stated that the burning of seacoles should be banned in favour of brushwood or charcoal. However, due the economic benefits brought about in industry by the efficiency of burning coals, this was ignored. The stench of the fumes did lead to its use being banned around Westminster, and at the Tower of London at specified times, with the aim of locating coal burning industries away from the Royal palaces, though in the early 17th century brewers at Westminster were admonished for burning seacole there. By this juncture, the rise in the burning of coal and its spread to the domestic setting was of sufficient concern for John Evelyn (Fig. 72) to publish his study *Fumifugium; or the Inconvenience of the Air and Smoke of London Dissipated* in 1661, an essay that remains highly relevant today (Fig. 73). In this, he observes that,

> This cloud is so inextricably mixed with the naturally wholesome and excellent air that the inhabitants can breathe nothing but thick, dirty, smoggy air. This makes them vulnerable to thousands of diseases, so that catarrh, coughs and tuberculosis are more prevalent in this city than any other in the world. I shall not here describe at length the nature of smoke or emissions which vary in respect to the different materials being burnt, for they are generally known to be noxious and unhealthy. However, what is certain is that, of all the common and familiar materials that emit pollution, the excessive demand for, and use of, sea coal in the city of London exposes it to one of the foulest criticisms and reproaches that can be aimed at such a noble, and otherwise incomparably magnificent city... The problem is caused by the works of the brewers, dyers, lime-burners, salt and soap boilers, and other private trades; the emissions from a single one of these evidently pollutes the air more than all of London's chimneys put together.

Following this, in 1662, John Gaunt produced an analysis of mortality in the City in his pamphlet *Natural and Political Observations... Made upon the Bills of Mortality*, suggesting that air pollution caused by the burning of coal was causing a significant problem to public health in London.

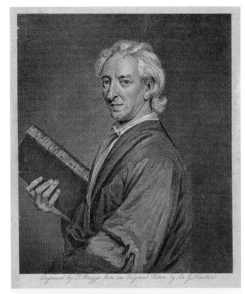

Figure 72 John Evelyn
(Wellcome Images)

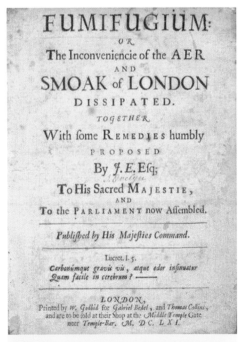

Figure 73 Frontispiece of *Fumifugium* by John Evelyn, 1661
(public domain)

Industrial London: black hair, black whiskers, black soup

Although the large factories of the north were absent, the booming manufacturing industries in the City were heavily reliant on the rapidly developing powered technologies. Pivotal to this race for production efficiency was coal (Fig. 74). Coal provided the means to power steam engines for ships and omnibuses and to fuel machines and power stations. Furthermore, it was not only a source of heat but also one of light. The Gas Light and Coke Company converted coal into coal gas which was then used to fuel gas-jet lamps, first appearing on Westminster Bridge in 1807. Leigh's *New Picture of London* of 1830 states that The City Gas Company consumed 9000 chaldrons of coals [per annum] (approximately 12,600 imperial tons), and lit about 8000 lamps via 50 miles (80.5 km) of pipes. The acquisition, trade and provision of coal became ever more critical as coal use in London grew rapidly.

According to Henry Mayhew, only one or two ships were needed to meet the supply of coal required to the City in 1550. By 1848, this figure had increased to 12,267

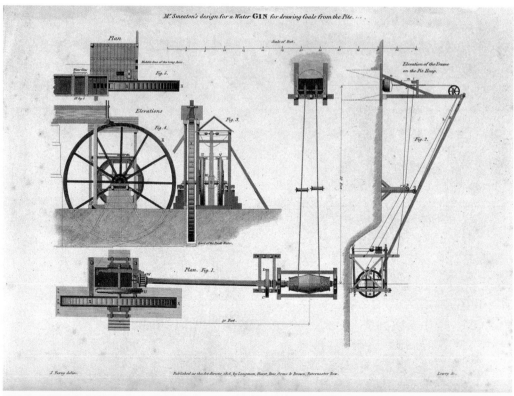

Figure 74 Machinery designed by Smeaton for extracting coal from the pits. Etching by W. Lowry after J. Farey, 1816
(Wellcome Images)

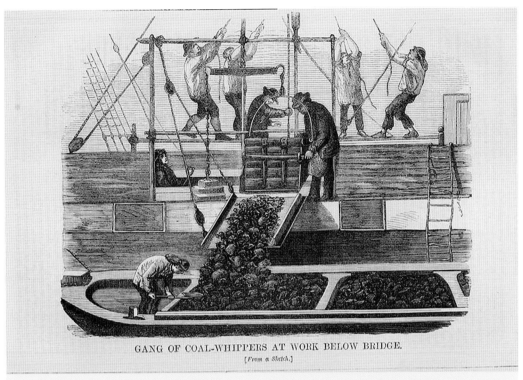

Figure 75 Illustration of coal-whippers from Henry Mayhew's *London Labour and the London Poor*, 1861
(cc-by-sa/2.0 https://www.flickr.com/photos/internetarchivebookimages/14577158380)

cargoes carried by 2177 ships (Table 5), employing approximately 21,600 sailors in addition to 4000 coal labourers and 4000 coal-whippers and porters (Fig. 75).

At this time, it was estimated that the coal fields of Great Britain ran to approximately 9000 square miles (23,310 km², producing 32 million tons of coal annually. Approximately one-third of this supply went to the iron-works, 8,500,000 tons was shipped coast wise, 2,500,000 tons was exported and the remaining third was used inland. Four million tons of coal was brought to London in 1848 and at that time, half a million tons was used by the gas work.

By definition, the coal industry was a dirty business. Coal dust saturated every aspect of the environment. 'All about the ship partakes of the grimness of the prevailing hue. The sails are black, the gilding on the figurehead of the vessel becomes

Table 5 Coal ships and Cargoes coming into London Port (after Mayhew 1861)

Date	No. of ships*/cargoes	Tons
1550	2	–
1615	200*	–
1705	600*	–
1805	4856	1,350,000
1820	5884	1,692,992
1830	7108	2,079,275
1840	9132	2,566,899
1845	11987	3,403,320
1848	2177*/12,267	3,418,340

blackened ... the workers have black hair and black whiskers, no matter what the original hue. It is a jest ... that everything is black in a collier, especially the soup' noted Mayhew in the 1840s. The work of coal-whipping, or hauling the coal out of the hold of a ship onto the docks, was long, hot and arduous work, often in the cramped conditions of the ship's hull, ridden with coal dust (Fig. 76). It would have been constantly inhaled during the working day. On average, 98 tons of coal, or 1568 baskets full, was shifted a day between a gang of nine men, manually lifted and carried 23–30 ft (7–9 m) up out of the hold. One coal-heaver explained that he had to carry 298 lb (135 kg) of coal on his back up a vertical ladder of 35 steps – and that the work was such a physical strain that it was common practice to put a piece of coal in your mouth to stop yourself biting your tongue when gritting your teeth to get through the effort.

Not only was the inhalation of coal dust at work perpetual but the accommodation that workers endured, especially those single men working under a publican, was cramped, overcrowded and poorly ventilated, with bed-linen changed only once a fortnight. On top of this, the tap-rooms in pubs were also small, dark, dirty, crowded

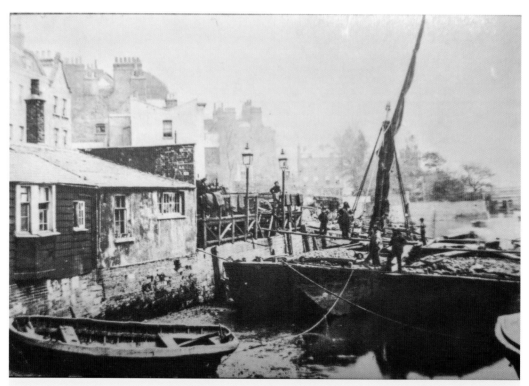

Figure 76 Coal barges, Chelsea Reach, 1860s
(public domain)

and ill-ventilated, often so thick with tobacco smoke that it wasn't possible to see through the murky air. Despite working on the dockside, clean air was not plentiful. Even the view along the river is described by Mayhew as a 'forest of masts in the distance and ... tall chimneys vomiting clouds of black smoke'. With plumes of smoke also rising from row after row of terraced house chimneys, London was said by *The Spectator* in 1889 to be in a 'reign of darkness' so that its inhabitants lived 'in something not far from perpetual twilight'.

Other trades that suffered similar effects of dust inhalation in the City would have been the carpenters and cabinet makers, the foundries, the textile industry, brick and tile making and the pottery industry, all of which generated fine dust inhaled by 'dust-coloured' workers, in similarly ill-ventilated and cramped surroundings. Often, piece work was undertaken at home in poor quality housing that was equally airless. Many of these trades were in the East End, especially in Bethnal Green, Spitalfields and Bow.

London's Great Smog

Despite the efforts of the Coal Smoke Abatement Society founded in 1898, the failure to tackle air pollution from coal burning in the domestic, commercial and public transport sectors, in favour of the economic success it brought, continued to lead to rapidly deteriorating air quality in the City (Fig. 77).

This culminated in the toxic 'Great Smog of London' descending upon the city on the 5 December 1952, resulting from a combination of cold weather, an anticyclone and the collection of fossil fuel smoke particles (Figs 78 and 79). Sulphur dioxide levels rose to five or six times above normal with some areas peaking at ten times the normal levels. The outcome was fatal, leading to the deaths of between 4000 and 12,000 people, with 100,000 more suffering illness of the respiratory tract. This finally led to passing of the Clean Air Act 1956. An increased awareness of the direct impact on the environment of coal

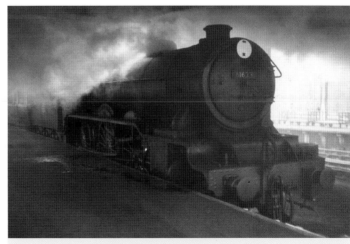

Figure 77 Liverpool Street Station, 1952
(cc-by-sa/2.0 https://www.flickr.com/photos/16179216@N07)

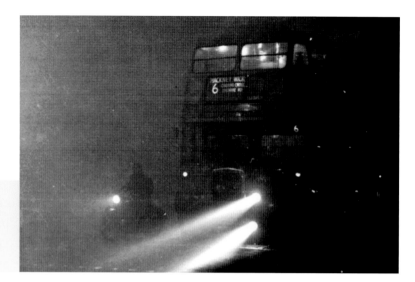

Figure 78 Police motorcycle escort to guide a bus through the smog in London, 1952

(Alan Farrow, https://www.flickr.com/photos/116071498@N08, Public Domain, Mark 1.0)

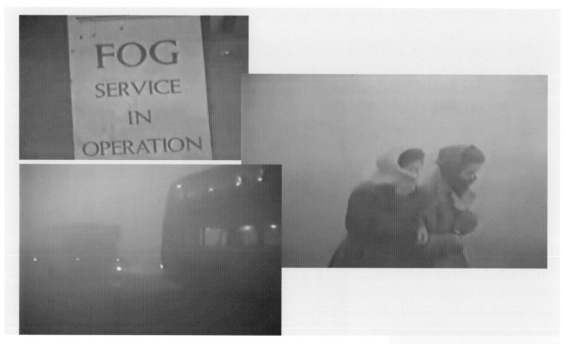

Figure 79 Stills from footage of the 1952 Great Smog of London

burning and traffic fumes has provided the impetus to improve our air quality, leading to technological shifts in transport, energy usage and even wearing face masks. However, these issues remain controversial, with some disputing the scientific evidence for the impact of these pollutants, claiming that this period is just another temporary shift in the long trajectory of the planet's environmental history.

Registration of the cause of death prior to 1837 was not consistently undertaken and even from this date, descriptions and classifications have changed over time according to the rapid development of medicine. So how can we really tell if airborne irritants and diseases of the lungs have increased with industrialisation? Was London really a hotspot compared to the rest of the country? Can we identify early trends in smoking prior to the earliest documentary records and assess its impact?

Affects of lung disease on the human skeleton

Analysis of human skeletal remains can give us an insight into the history of chronic lung diseases due to changes we can see on the inside (visceral) surfaces of the ribs. This is where the pleura (lining of the lungs and the chest wall) is in contact with the ribs (Fig. 80).

If affected by a chronic inflammatory condition, the inflamed pleura thicken and can cause new bone formation on the visceral surfaces of the ribs. These are known as 'visceral surface rib lesions' (VSRLs) (Fig. 81). This reaction to the bone is non-specific, i.e. it can be caused by numerous inflammatory lung illnesses, so it is not possible to make a specific diagnosis from the presence of VSRLs in the skeleton alone. They are best equated with the clinical diagnosis of chronic pleurisy, which has many causes. These include viral, bacterial and fungal infections as well as certain autoimmune and inherited disorders and, in some cases, lung cancer.

Some osteological investigations have found that up to 70% of VSRLs are associated with tuberculosis and although tuberculosis is a known clinical cause of pleurisy, clinical evidence for VSRLs is rare since they can only be observed on dry bone. Additionally, not all chronic cases of lung diseases will result in VSRLs. What we can say is that when VSRLs are present in human skeletal remains, the individual has suffered chronic inflammation of the lungs. When we look at bone changes in the human skeleton it is often not possible to tell if these pathologies caused the death of the individual. Pathological data from human skeletal remains is therefore considered to reflect illness (morbidity) rather than cause of death (mortality).

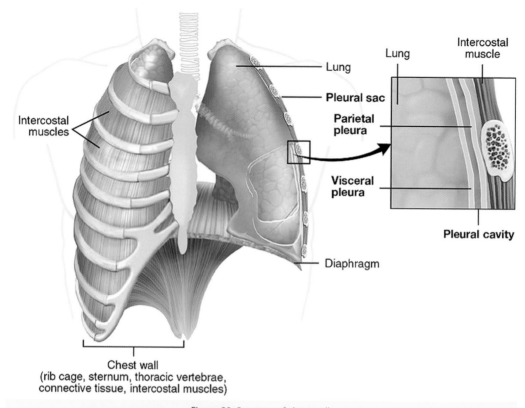

Lung

Pleural sac

Parietal pleura

Visceral pleura

Diaphragm

Intercostal muscles

Lung

Intercostal muscle

Pleural cavity

Chest wall
(rib cage, sternum, thoracic vertebrae,
connective tissue, intercostal muscles)

Figure 80 Structure of chest wall

(Open Stax College, cc-by-sa/4.0, http://cnx.org/content/col11496/1.6/)

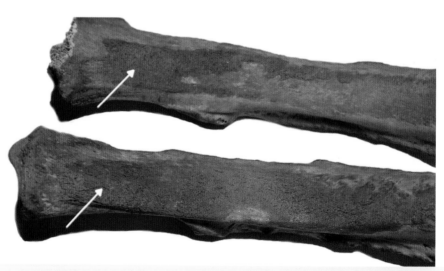

Figure 81 Visceral surface rib lesions (VSRLs) consist of bone formation on the inner surfaces of the ribs, seen here as dark brown deposits of new bone on top of the normal light brown rib surface (arrowed), Upton-on-Severn, Worcestershire

(Ossafreelance)

Evidence for visceral surface rib lesions

In total, we looked at the human skeletal remains of 1325 individuals excavated from archaeological sites dating to the Industrial period, whose skeletons were more than 70% complete and were well preserved. This ensured that at least some of the ribs were present and could be observed for the presence of visceral surface rib lesions (VSRLs). A further 1028 individuals of the same level of completeness and preservation were also included in a sample of individuals dating to the pre-Industrial period, for comparison. Both the samples comprised skeletal assemblages from within and from non-metropolitan areas outside London.

In the pre-Industrial period rates of VSRLs were low. Only 13, or 2.9%, of the 456 individuals analysed from pre-Industrial London had chronic inflammatory lung diseases (Table 6). This rate was quite similar to the 1.6% of the 572 individuals affected outside of London (Table 8). In the Industrial period, however, it was clear from the skeletal evidence that things were very different. While the rate of VSRLs had risen slightly to 4.2% among those 526 individuals examined from outside of London (Table 9), a huge increase was seen in the London population. Of the 799

Table 6 Incidence of VSRLs in pre-Industrial London

	n	N	%
St Mary Graces	0	31	0
Billingsgate	0	11	0
Broadgate	3	36	8.3
Spitalfields (14)	10	378	2.6
Total	13	456	2.9

N= total number of individuals and
n= number of individuals affected

Table 7 Incidence of VSRLs in Industrial London

Site	n	N	%
New Covent Garden, Nine Elms	1	19	5.3
St. Bride's Crypt	8	94	8.5
Mare Street	11	130	8.5
Chelsea Old Church	5	43	11.6
Bow Baptists	32	144	22.2
Lower St Bride's	26	103	25.2
Bethnal Green	73	266	27.4
Total	156	799	19.5

Table 9 Incidence of VSRLs in Industrial non-metropolitan areas

	n	N	%
Barton-upon-Humber	1	84	1.2
Brentford	9	103	8.7
Coach Lane	0	42	0
Fewston	5	30	16.7
Holy Trinity Stratford	1	14	7.1
Upton on Severn	2	11	18.2
Wharram Percy	0	22	0
Swinton	1	48	2.1
Hereford Cathedral Close	3	172	1.7
Total	22	526	4.2

Table 8 Incidence of VSRLs in pre-Industrial non-metropolitan areas

	n	N	%
Barton-upon-Humber	1	156	0.6
Holy Trinity Stratford	0	19	0
Wharram Percy	0	114	0
Hereford 1	4	173	2.3
Hereford Cathedral Close	4	110	3.6
Total	9	572	1.6

individuals in the London industrial sample, 156 had VSRLs, indicating a significant rise in chronic inflammatory lung conditions from 2.9% to 19.5% (Table 7).

The huge increase in chronic lung diseases during the Industrial period was not uniformly present across the City. The area with the highest prevalence rate of VSRLs was Bethnal Green (27.4%) whereas New Covent Garden (Nine Elms) had the lowest (5.3%). Nine Elms at this time still retained its open, green areas used for market gardening in contrast to Bethnal Green which, during the Industrial period, became a very built-up, populous suburban area of terraced housing, being located closer to the central City. Numbers in the area grew from 1800 in 1743 to 16,430 by 1871. It was noted that, by 1826, there was little open space between settlements and by this time, several factories had been established here, replacing the former market gardening economy.

The effects of our living environments within the City

This stark difference in the local environments within London may well have played a very important role in the prevalence of chronic inflammatory lung diseases. To investigate this further, we examined the prevalence of VSRLs from skeletal assemblages known to originate from areas of high social status (Table 10) with improved living conditions in comparison to assemblages from low social status areas (Table 11) with poorer housing and environmental conditions. The high status assemblages consisted of Chelsea Old Church, St Bride's Crypt, Fleet Street and Mare Street, Hackney. The low status assemblages were from Bow, the lower churchyard of St Bride's, Fleet Street and Bethnal Green. We discovered a significant difference between the prevalence rates of the two groups, with evidence for chronic lung inflammation being almost three times higher in the low social status group (25.5%) than that of the high status group (9.0%).

Many people living in the East End areas and the central area around Farringdon lived in overcrowded, meagre and often squalid conditions (Fig. 82). The expansion of housing was rapid. Between 1839 and 1848, Henry Mayhew estimated that 200 miles (over 320 km) of new streets had been built in London with no less than 6405 new houses constructed annually, all heated by burning coal or wood. Bethnal Green was said to be three times as crowded as the rest of London with 17 houses per acre compared to an average of 5.5 (Fig.

Table 10 Incidence of VSRLs at high status sites

	n	N	%
Chelsea Old Church	5	43	11.6
St Bride's Crypt	8	94	8.5
Mare Street Hackney	11	130	8.5
Total	24	267	9.0

Table 11 Incidence of VSRLs at low status sites

	n	N	%
Bow Baptists	32	144	22.2
Lower St Bride's	26	103	25.2
Bethnal Green	73	266	27.4
Total	131	513	25.5

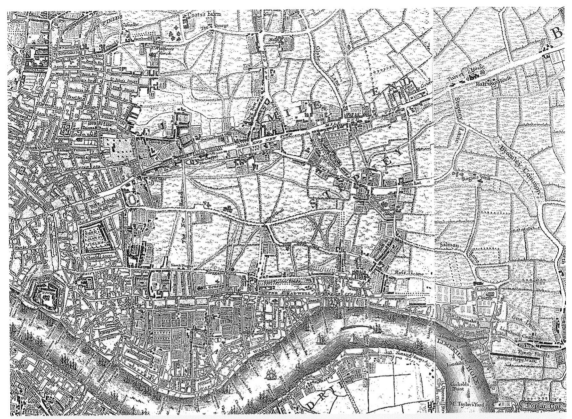

Figure 82 John Rocque's *Exact Survey of the Citys of London Westminster ye Borough of Southwark and the Country near Town Mile Round* illustrating the open fields of the East End in 1741–1745

(Birkbeck History Dept. https://commons.wikimedia.org/wiki/File:1745_Roque_Map.jpg, public domain, CCO)

83). In the 1840s the housing situation here was dire, described as 'more huts than houses, built in swamps, at cheap rent'. Nowhere else in London were so many low-rented houses to be found, 93% rated at under £20. Most houses constructed since 1800 were of two storeys, without foundations, small and damp, made from the cheapest timber and half-fired bricks with badly pitched roofs, 'erected by speculative builders of the most scampy class'. This occurred to a certain extent because of the medieval 'copyhold' status of land in the East End, a system that ensured short leaseholds only, preventing investment in large scale development. This poor quality of housing impacted severely on health status, especially regarding chronic lung conditions, since the home provided not only a living space but also a place of work (Fig. 84).

Individuals from Chelsea Old Church, St Bride's Crypt and Mare Street, Hackney are all known to have been wealthy, living in superior areas of London in better quality housing (Fig. 85). Chelsea had also initially been a relatively open and green area, Jonathan Swift commenting in his diary in May 1711: 'that about our town we

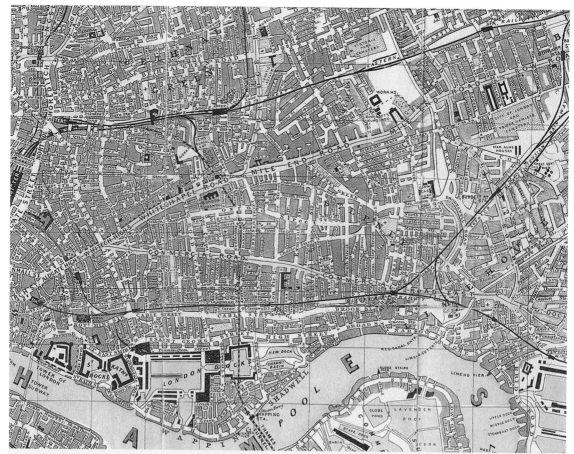

Figure 83 1882 Reynolds *Map of the East End*, depicting the dense network of streets and housing that replaced the open areas
(Birkbeck History Dept, https://commons.wikimedia.org/wiki/File:1882_Reynolds_Map.jpg, public domain, CCO)

are mowing already and making hay, and it smells so sweet as we walk through the flowery meads'. There was poor quality housing in Chelsea and Hackney but it existed side by side with some much more impressive and larger residences frequented by the individuals in our high status assemblages. This is a pattern of habitation that is seen throughout the City's occupation since the early medieval period, with the wealthy City dwellers living cheek-by-jowl with poorer citizens. Over time, however, as villages and towns became submerged by suburban development, individual districts within London evolved to become much more distinct from one another in terms of wealth, class and living environment. In the 1830s in Chelsea, over half of the housing was considered to be 4th class (mid-point in the range of housing quality categorisation) and, by the 1870s, even grander new houses were being built for rich people with artistic inclinations. Similarly, by the 1880s, residents in Mare Street, Hackney were described as 'well-to-do'.

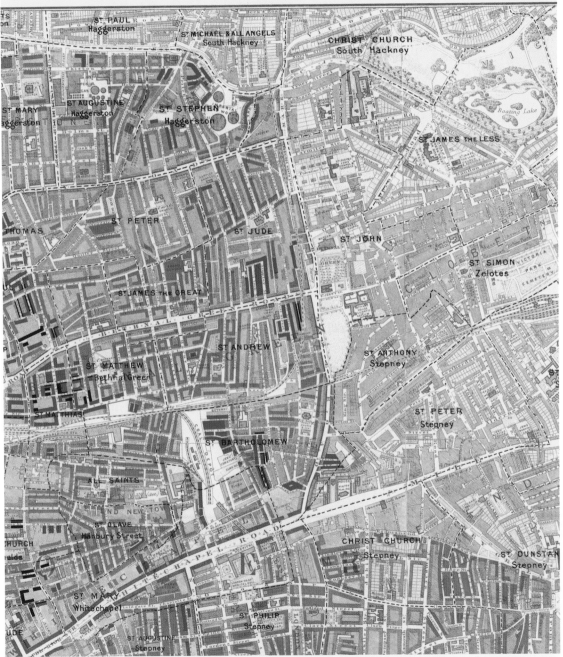

MAP DESCRIPTIVE OF LONDON POVERTY, 1898-9
(IN 12 SHEETS)

Figure 84 1899 Spitalfields and Bethnal Green area on Charles Booth's map of poverty

(https://booth.lse.ac.uk/learn-more/download-maps, public domain, Mark 1.0)

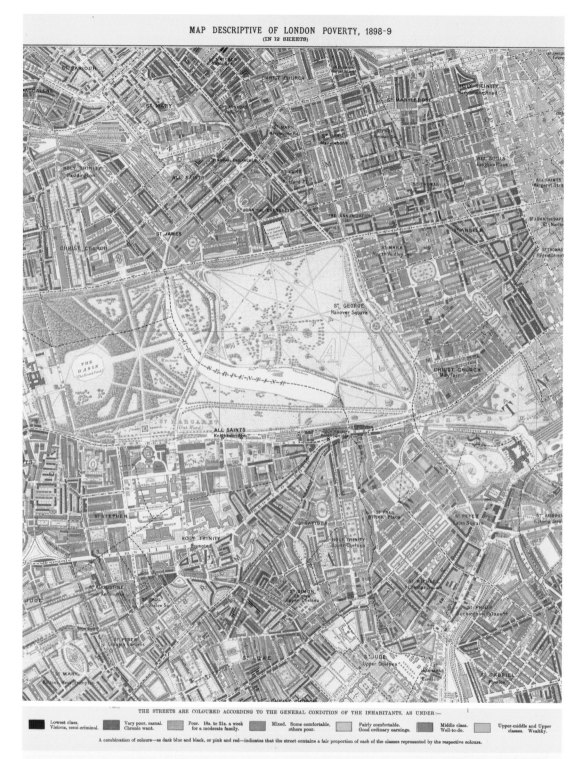

MAP DESCRIPTIVE OF LONDON POVERTY, 1898-9

(IN 12 SHEETS)

THE STREETS ARE COLOURED ACCORDING TO THE GENERAL CONDITION OF THE INHABITANTS, AS UNDER:—

Lowest class. Vicious, semi-criminal. | Very poor, casual. Chronic want. | Poor. 18s. to 21s. a week for a moderate family. | Mixed. Some comfortable, others poor. | Fairly comfortable. Good ordinary earnings. | Middle class. Well-to-do. | Upper-middle and Upper classes. Wealthy.

A combination of colours—as dark blue and black, or pink and red—indicates that the street contains a fair proportion of each of the classes represented by the respective colours.

Figure 85 1899 Chelsea area on Charles Booth's map of poverty (https://booth.lse.ac.uk/learn-more/download-maps, public domain, Mark 1.0.) Key: yellow: Upper middle and upper classes. Wealthy; red: Middle class, well-to-do; light blue: Poor, 18s to 21s a week for a moderate family; dark blue: Very poor, casual, chronic want; black: Lowest class ... occasional labourers, street sellers, loafers, criminals and semi-criminals

Differences between men and women, young and old

We found that in the populations outside of London and in the pre-industrial population of London, there was little difference between prevalence rates of VSRLs between males and females (Fig. 86). However, there was a significant difference between rates of VSRLs in males and females in the London industrial population, indicating an increased exposure of males, particularly those of young and

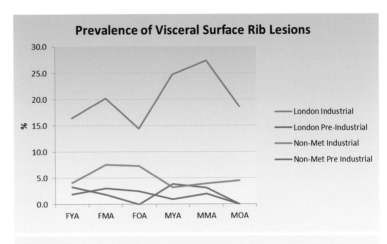

Figure 86 Prevalence rates of VSRLs in female (F) and male (M) adults according to age (YA = young adult, MA = middle adult and OA = old adult)

middle adult age, to chronic inflammatory lung conditions than females. This suggests that young and middle aged males in the industrialised City occupied environments or were engaged in behaviours that were more hazardous to their health in terms of inhaling polluted air compared to females.

The disparity between the sexes in rates of VSRLs is likely to be due to a large part to differences in working environments experienced by men and women at this time, especially in the case of lower status individuals (Fig. 87). Overall, 29.5% of low status males had VSRLs compared to 11.2% of high status males. We also found that 82.6% of the 87 males with VSRLs in our socially stratified industrial London sample were of low social status. Although rates of VSRLs in females were significantly lower than males in industrial London, the same effect of social status was found within the female group: 86.8% of the 68 females in the sample of individuals

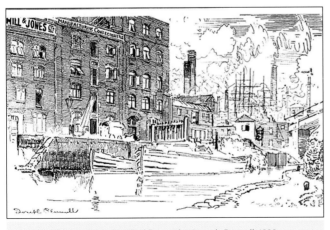

Figure 87 An East End Factory by Joseph Pennell, 1899
(Jacqueline Banerjee, The Victorian Web, http://www.victorianweb.org/)

with VSRLs were low status, with a rate of 21.9% of VSRLs amongst all low status females compared to only 6.8% of all high status females. It is clear from this data that social status also has a major role to play in the prevalence rates of chronic inflammatory lung diseases.

'The hazy environs of "Smokiana"'

Since tobacco was brought into England from Italy in 1565 by Sir John Hawkins, London in particular, has had a special relationship with it. James I who, in a bid to regulate what he termed, 'a custom loathsome to the eye, hateful to the nose, harmful to the brain, dangerous to the lungs', decreed in 1619 that tobacco could only be imported into London and pipes could only be manufactured by makers under Royal Charter in Westminster. This, however, was a short-lived campaign and in 1634 Charles I rebranded the group *The Tobacco-pipe Makers of London and Westminster and England and Wales*. Today the group is known as the *Worshipful Company of Tobacco Pipe Makers and Tobacco Blenders* and is still based in the City. Tobacco smoking caught on fast and, by the 1840s, London Dock housed tobacco warehouses that alone covered 5 acres (2 ha). Tobacco could be consumed by pipesmoking, snorting snuff, smoking hand rolled cigars and finally, after 1883 following the invention of the Bonsack machine, by smoking the newly mass manufactured and much cheaper cigarettes.

Up to the late Victorian period smoking was largely a habit of the male domain. Smoking by females was seen as a vulgar habit, associated with prostitution. Conversely, smoking became a pursuit of intellectualism for higher status males, often gathering in social clubs to

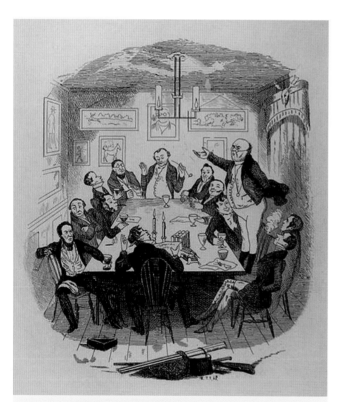

Figure 88 *Mr. Pickwick addresses the club* from *The Writings of Charles Dickens*, volume 1, 1894 (R. Seymour)

discuss the latest bourgeois ideals and current affairs while lighting up (Fig. 88). Tobacco shops sprang up all over London (Fig. 89). In the low status setting, pipe smoking was much more associated with hospitality and communality. Free clay pipes were provided at Inns for smokers, for example.

Pipes varied in size and shape over time and according to trends in their usage. Later clay pipes dating to the 18th century tended to have a larger bowl for holding more tobacco than earlier versions and in the mid-18th century, pipes with very long stems c. 450–600 mm in length known as 'aldermans' or 'straws' (Fig. 90), were introduced for 'leisure smoking', allowing a gentleman to hold the bowl comfortably while seated, perhaps in what is now commonly known as a 'smoker's bow chair'. In comparison, labourers used 'cuttys' or 'nose warmers' (Fig. 91). These had very short stems, often squared off so that they could be gripped between the teeth, leaving the hands free to carry on working.

Evidence for smoking in its earliest period is present in the skeleton in the form of pipe smoking notches (Fig. 92). These are grooves worn into the anterior teeth from their habitual use to grip the clay pipe stem. Therefore, although these grooves provide evidence for smoking, it is restricted to the long-

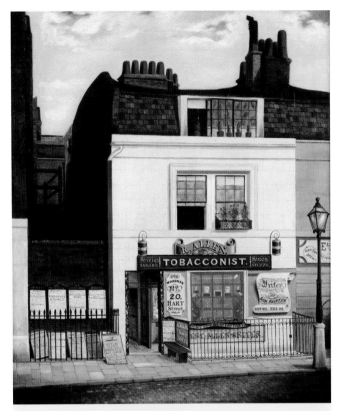

Figure 89 Tobacconist shop
(© Museum of London)

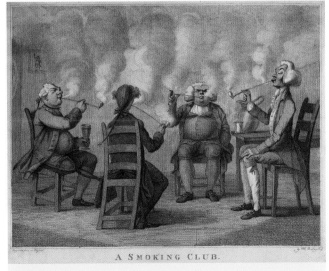

A SMOKING CLUB.

Figure 90 *Four Georgian gentlemen sit in their club seriously engaged in smoking Alderman pipes.* Engraving with stipple by H. Bunbury, 1794
(Wellcome Collection. cc-by/4.0)

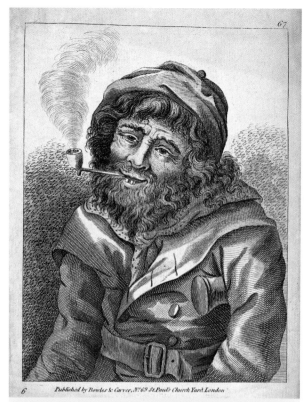

Figure 91 *A seated man in a double-breasted coat smoking a short stem 'Cutty' pipe while he rests on a crutch under his left arm.* Line engraving with etching. London (No. 69 St Paul's Church Yard) Bowles & Carver

term use of clay pipes only. Tar staining on teeth can often also be observed on inside (lingual) surfaces of teeth but is most often associated with the presence of grooves and only appears rarely in isolation. The rates of smoking as detected by analysis of human skeletal remains should, therefore, be considered a minimum estimate.

We examined a sample of 922 individuals, all of whom had at least half their anterior dentition and ribs present, to investigate smoking rates in London and non-metropolitan populations based outside of London and its relationship with the presence of visceral surface rib lesions to assess any association with chronic inflammatory lung diseases. Evidence for smoking rates were consistent between the Londoners (11.6%) and non-Londoners (10.4%). Also consistent was the predominance of the presence of pipesmoking notches in males (19.7% in the City and 16.4% outside of London) compared to females (2.5% in the City and 3.7% outside of London), irrespective of their geographical location. Of the total 115 smokers, only 13.0% were females. There was no relationship between age at death and the presence of pipesmoking grooves amongst either males or females. Interestingly, no significant relationship was found between social status and smoking among males, though the percentage of smokers among low status males was slightly higher (22.2%) compared to high status males (15.1%).

The mortality profiles of both smokers and non-smokers were compared to investigate if smoking produced higher numbers of deaths of younger male individuals compared to the non-smokers. No evidence of any impact on mortality was found (Fig. 93). Looking more closely at the data for the industrial London males, we found that any differences in the mortality age profiles between smokers and non-smokers was explained by their social status (Figs 94 and 95). Once social status

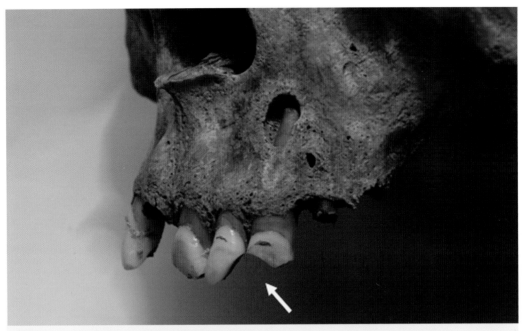

Figure 92 Pipe smoking grooves, male, Upton-upon-Severn, non-metropolitan Industrial
(Ossafreelance)

was taken into account, mortality age profiles between smokers and non-smokers mirrored each other very closely.

No significant relationship was found between smoking and the presence of rib lesions. This reflects the medical observation that smoking itself does not cause pleurisy. However, what is clinically observed is that smoking will exacerbate any pre-existing lung inflammation. As we have already seen, social status was important in the presence of rib lesions due to the unhealthy environments and noxious airs of lower status living and working areas within the City. We found similar trends within the smoking group. For example, of the 16 male smokers with rib lesions, 93.8% were low status and low status males who smoked were significantly more likely to have rib lesions than high status smokers. However, the same was true of low status male non-smokers compared to their high status counterparts. It is possible then, that smoking during this period exacerbated cases of chronic lung inflammation but overall, was much less significant than the generally dire, smoky and dust ridden environmental conditions that low status individuals were exposed to. Furthermore, amongst the higher status groups, non-smokers had higher rates of VSRL's than smokers, suggesting that even those of wealthier means did not entirely escape the environmental effects of living in London's polluted air.

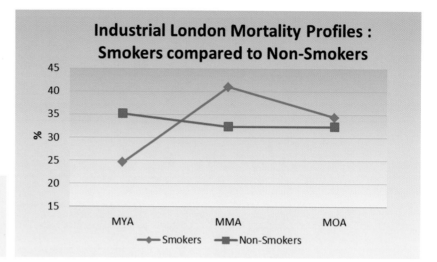

Figure 93 Mortality profiles smokers compared to non-smokers, Industrial London

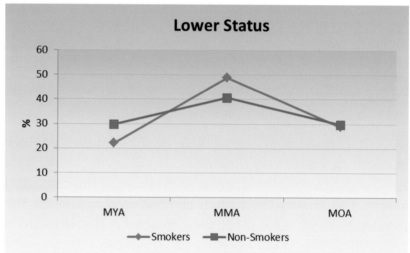

Figure 94 Mortality profiles for lower status smokers compared to non-smokers, Industrial London

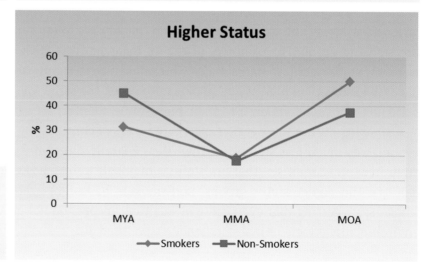

Figure 95 Mortality profiles for higher status smokers compared to non-smokers, Industrial London

Infections

Tuberculosis is well recognised as a disease of poverty, common in the overcrowded areas of city environments, causing wasting, fatigue, shortness of breath, coughing up blood and finally death. Nonetheless, in the Victorian period, the disease was heavily romanticised, as it caused the faces of its sufferers to look pale, delicate and, apparently, as interesting as some of the notable authors who died of the disease, such as D. H. Lawrence.

Recent research suggests that people are more likely to become infected with tuberculosis if they are also exposed to smoke. This includes smoke from burning wood and coal as well as active and passive cigarette smoking. Smoke particles clog up specialist immune cells called macrophages, our first line of defence against such infections, so that they are unable to function normally. Inhaling any kind of smoke, therefore, suppresses the immune system's ability to resist tuberculosis infection.

Historical data from the mortality records of 1851–1860 (Fig. 96) indicate that respiratory TB was differentiated from other diseases of the lungs as a cause of death, though it is not clear how accurately this was done. 'Respiratory tuberculosis' is notably a disease of young and middle aged adults compared to 'lung diseases', which predominantly affected old age adults. The consistency of the different age profiles for deaths caused by 'respiratory tuberculosis' and 'lung diseases' in both London and non-metropolitan populations demonstrates that the two separate causes of death were being recorded similarly by medical practitioners across the country. Unfortunately, this does not preclude misdiagnosis in some cases.

What we notice in the age profile of Industrial period London adults with visceral rib lesions is that young and middle adults are also more frequently affected than old adults. At first glance, this could be an indication that tuberculosis was a factor in the much higher rates of inflammatory lung diseases in London.

However, what is also evident is that mortality

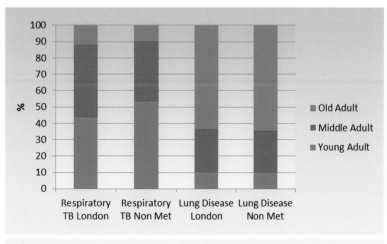

Figure 96 Age profile of respiratory TB cases and lung disease in adults from Mortality Records, 1851–1860

rates of respiratory tuberculosis were actually very similar in London (32.4%) and non-metropolitan (33.6%) young and middle aged adult populations. Despite the similar mortality rates of tuberculosis both in and outside of London, these two groups had very different rates of VSRLs (21.6% compared to 4.4%), indicating that young and middle aged Londoners experienced much higher rates of chronic inflammatory lung diseases than those outside the City. A similar pattern emerges examining the data for death by lung diseases in old adults: 20.7% of old age Londoners were recorded as having died due to lung diseases compared to 14.5% outside of London, whereas the disparity between the two groups in terms of VSRLs is much greater, at 16.6% compared to 3.6%.

The discrepancy between the two sets of data suggests that VSRLs are not reliable indicators of recorded respiratory tuberculosis mortality in past populations, most likely due to the fact that VSRLs are non-specific reactions and are multifactorial in aetiology, i.e., they can be caused by several different lung diseases. VSRLs also represent episodes of morbidity rather than mortality. For example, rib lesions in human skeletal remains can be active or healed, the latter indicating that the individual survived the period of lung inflammation. It is clear from the historical data that tuberculosis was a significant factor in the deaths of young and middle aged adults both in London and outside the City. However, despite the fact the age profiles of VSRLs and tuberculosis match in the London industrial population, we cannot infer any relationship between VSRLs and the presence of tuberculosis because of the disparity between the age profiles of VSRLs and tuberculosis outside of London. The same is also true of other 'lung diseases' in old age adults. Populations outside of London do not appear to have experienced chronic inflammatory lung diseases to the same extent as in the City. This is not to say that tuberculosis did not cause the increase in the VSRLs young to middle aged adult Londoners but that further, more specific, evidence, such as demonstrating the presence of TB through aDNA detection, is needed to prove the case. It seems likely, however, that the much higher rate of chronic inflammatory lung diseases in London was, at least in part, caused by air pollution, occupational dust, smoking and poorly ventilated living and working environments.

Pneumoconiosis

A significant risk to health from breathing-in polluted air is pneumoconiosis, which refers to lung disease caused by the inhalation of dust and its retention in the lungs. It is classified as an occupational disease and clinically, the condition has four subgroups based on the type of dust: coal worker's pneumoconiosis (Black Lung Disease), asbestosis, silicosis and other unspecified pneumoconiosis. It is common in people exposed to mineral dusts for long periods of time and is exacerbated by tobacco smoking. Although a minor form of the disease called anthracosis is found to some degree in most urban dwellers as a result of air pollution, pneumoconiosis represents a more serious condition. Symptoms include shortness of breath, coughing and chest tightness. The condition can cause lung inflammation, fibrosis and pleural effusion. In the 1940s, pneumoconiosis associated with coal dust was the most common occupational lung disease. In fact, silicosis is currently the most common occupational lung disease worldwide. However, the condition is rare in the UK. According to The Health and Occupation Reporting Network, in 2014, only 251 males were diagnosed with pneumoconiosis. No cases were found amongst females.

Medical research has demonstrated that there is an inter-relationship between silicosis and pulmonary tuberculosis. Individuals either with silicosis or having been exposed to silica over the duration of time are approximately four times more likely to contract pulmonary TB on average and this likelihood increases according to the severity of the silicosis present. The interaction between the two conditions is now recognised by a diagnosis of 'silicotuberculosis', where tuberculosis is contracted after having silicosis. Its onset can be delayed until after the exposure to occupational dust has ceased, indicating that chronic exposure to dust, especially at a younger age, creates a lifelong increased risk of pulmonary disease. Primary research into why silica increases the risk of tuberculosis suggests that the silica dust alters the immune response of the lungs, compromising the function of the immune cells (macrophages) responsible for destroying pathogens, in this case tuberculous mycobacteria. Given the increased air pollution in London in the past and the significantly increased VSRLs present in industrial populations in the City, particularly in low status males, it is probable that occupational respiratory diseases such as pneumoconiosis and silicotuberculosis contributed towards this raised level of chronic inflammatory lung disease. Thomas Frye, the works manager at Messrs Crowther and Weatherby's pottery factory in Bow, for example, is noted to have suffered ill health after 15 years of working at the furnaces on his porcelain experiments, and to have died of tuberculosis 3 years later in 1762.

More recently, asbestosis has been identified as the most common underlying cause of occupational lung cancer, though silicosis is also known to be a contributory factor. Approximately 9% of the population globally suffer from occupational lung cancer, 15% in men and 5% in women on average. In the UK, the construction sector has the highest rates of occupational cancer cases and deaths, mainly comprising lung cancer and mesothelioma from exposure to asbestos and silica.

Air pollution today

Many infectious diseases that were common during the Industrial period have been much reduced in rates in modern populations, thanks to the discovery and development of antibiotics and vaccines, as well as improved living conditions. Although, without treatment, infectious diseases such as tuberculosis are still a significant threat to health, they are not currently present as epidemic or endemic diseases in the UK. For example, the average rate of tuberculosis in England and Wales in 2013–5 was 12.0 per 100,000 (0.012%), a huge reduction from the mortality rates of 16–20% for respiratory tuberculosis recorded in adults of all age groups during the Industrial period. In epidemiology, the vast reduction of infectious disease leading to a significant shift towards new types of disease dominating human health in a population is known as a pathocenosis. The beginning of the 20th century and the medical revolution of this period represent a pathocenosis in the evolution of UK health, manifest as a transition from infectious to non-communicable diseases. Today, the most serious effects of air pollution on our health derive from anthropogenic factors rather than pathogens (Fig. 97).

Spatial distribution analysis of the data from Public Health England based on NHS Clinical Commissioning Group (CCG) data for their local areas from 2015–16

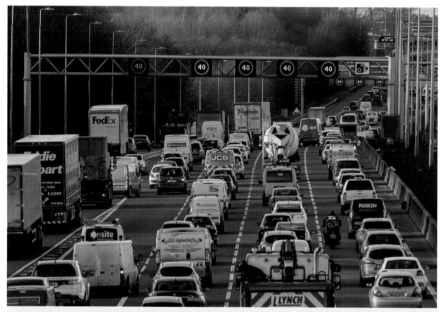

Figure 97 Traffic bottlenecks are strongly associated with high levels of anthropogenic air pollution
(Shutterstock.com)

illustrates that London still suffers the highest rates of mortality from anthropogenic air pollution in the country (6.3% of all-cause mortality). The data also indicate that the problem is not solely related to a rural or urban setting (Fig. 98). North Shields (North Tyneside CCG), the location of the Coach Lane burial ground, has the lowest rate of anthropogenic air pollution related mortality in our sample (3.5%), despite the wider area being more urban.

By comparison, towns of equal or even smaller size in fairly rural settings such as Hereford (Herefordshire CCG) (4.3%), Upton-on-Severn (South Worcestershire CCG)

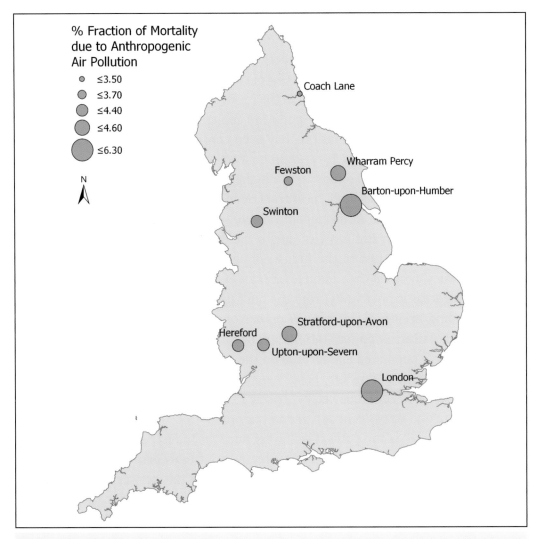

Figure 98 National statistics for percentage fraction of mortality due to anthropogenic air pollution (Public Health England, 2015–2016)

(4.4%) or Stratford-upon-Avon (South Warwickshire CCG) (4.6%), have slightly higher rates of mortality linked to air pollution. On the other hand, Swinton (Salford CCG), which is highly urban, has a relatively low rate of mortality related to air pollution (4.3%) while Barton-upon-Humber (NE Lincolnshire CCG) has a rate similar to outer London (5.7%). Clearly, the situation is complex and contributed to by several factors. This includes density of road traffic and bottlenecks, but also shipping and aviation, as well as density of habitation and the weather. Local industries across the country, such as waste incineration, which is set to expand, are also a threat to air quality. The metropolitan setting of London is not only the most populous but also has one of the densest transport networks in the UK. In 2019, a statement by the Committee on the Medical Effects of Air Pollutants (COMEAP) highlighted the excessive concentration of particulate pollution in London Underground stations, which is up to 30 times higher than roadside levels in the City. Also of concern is the recent trend towards the re-use of open fires and wood-burners in the residential setting. It has been estimated that 25–33% of London's particulate pollution comes from domestic fires today and, during a period of high air pollution, may even contribute up to half of particulate pollution in the City. These factors act in concert to exponentially increase the air pollution mortality rate in London to the highest in the country.

Within the City, areas located in central London north of the River Thames suffer with the highest levels of anthropogenic air pollution related mortality, despite the fact that these are high status areas, due to the density of road traffic and exhaust fumes (Fig. 99). In contrast to the Industrial period, the East end areas of London, such as Hackney, Bethnal Green and Bow enjoy reduced levels of air pollution, as is the case with areas located away from the built up suburbs and closer to more open areas, including Brentford, by now in outer London, and Nine Elms which, since the closure of Battersea power station, is now a much cleaner, inner city parkland area, less densely populated and located on the south bank of the river. Attempts to reduce traffic pollution in the City have been made by the introduction of the London Congestion Charge in 2003 followed by stricter regulation in 2019 by creating an Ultra Low Emission Zone across central London (Fig. 100).

Coal use in the UK is currently at its lowest since the Industrial period and with the concomitant contraction of the coal industry, rates of coalworkers' pneumoconiosis had fallen to 0.8% between 1998 and 2000, compared to 12% between 1959 and 1963. Silicosis was first recognised as an industrial disease in 1919 under the *Workmen's Compensation Acts*. Since then, occupational health surveillance and the improved regulation of working environments, including setting work-place exposure limits (WEL) for respirable crystalline silica (RCS) in industry, have had a significant impact

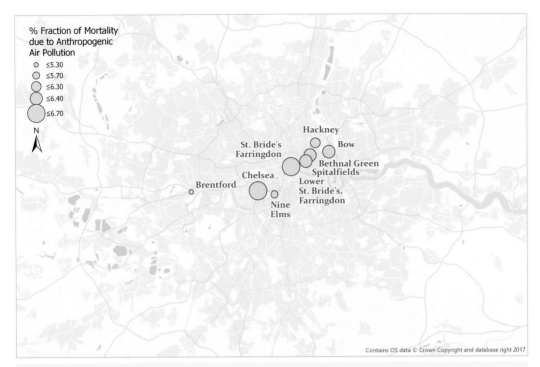

Figure 99 London statistics for percentage fraction of mortality due to anthropogenic air pollution (Public Health England, 2015–2016)

on the prevalence of occupational lung diseases. However, new sources of respiratory diseases are being discovered on a regular basis. There are now concerns regarding manufactured carbon nanotubes (MCNs) used in high frequency in electronic devices and accessories, such as printers, Li-on batteries and cables, and for industrial processing. Diacetyl (2,3-butanedione), a volatile butter-flavoured diketone (a chemical compound often used in food flavourings), has also been identified as the primary source of a number of serious cases of respiratory disease in the popcorn industry. An outbreak of lung illnesses also has occurred in workers involved in the manufacture of flat panel display screens caused by indium-tin oxide (ITO). Outside of manufacturing, the recent intensification of agriculture has also resulted in high exposures of endotoxins (bacteria, moulds and their toxins).

Almost half of agents or exposure circumstances identified as carcinogenic are occupational and most of these are respiratory carcinogens. Worryingly, however, it is estimated that only 2% of chemicals used in commerce have been tested sufficiently to identify if they are carcinogenic. Rates of recognised occupational respiratory disease are therefore set to rise and occupational asthma is now a chief

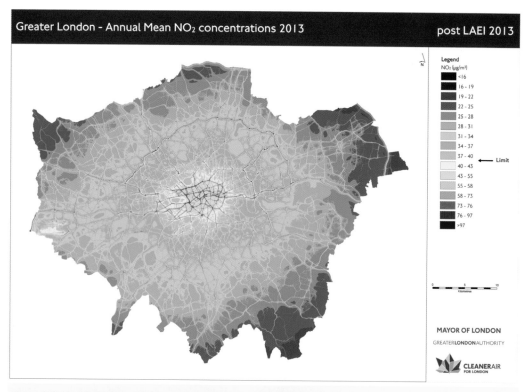

Figure 100 Modelled Mean NO2 air pollution, caused by motor vehicle exhaust fumes and burning fossil fuels, for 2013 (ug/m3). Arrow indicating the UK objective/EU limit for air quality limit

(London Datastore, Greater London Authority, London Atmospheric Emissions Inventory (LAEI) 2013 Concentration Maps)

health concern. The changing age demographic of the workforce may also lead to increasing rates in the future. People are staying in work longer or are returning to work at older ages, when they are more susceptible to lung infections. In addition, the regulation of work-places throughout Europe is now increasingly the responsibility of the employer rather than the state which, in the past, was not effective. For some, especially migrant workers who, because of their circumstances, may be forced to take low income jobs in the manufacturing industries, this may lead to increased risk of occupational diseases, not least because of a fear of reporting poor working conditions or a lack of access to health care.

The reduction of wider environmental causes of lung diseases linked to occupation, infectious disease and poor housing shone the spotlight on cigarette smoke as a major health concern during the late 20th century. Dramatically falling from its peak in the early 20th century, when smoking was actively promoted as a health benefit (Fig. 101) and was also enthusiastically taken up women as a symbol of liberation and equality, the national average estimate of smoking rates in 2015–6 was 18.1%.

This is similar to that observed in the industrial skeletal samples but includes all durations of smoking rather than only the long-term habit indicated by the presence of pipe-grooves worn into the teeth over a number of years. Modern rates of smoking in London and outside of London are the same (18.5%), reflecting the earlier trend found in the Industrial period. Within London, the highest smoking rate areas was City and Hackney (21.8%) followed closely by Tower Hamlets, East London (21.1%). The lowest was Central London (Westminster CCG) (16.2%). Outside of the City, the Barton-upon-Humber area (NE Lincolnshire CCG) reported the highest rate of smokers (23.8%) along with the Swinton area (Salford CCG) (23.0%). The lowest rates of smoking in non-metropolitan areas were found in the Stratford-upon-Avon area (South Warwickshire CCG) (14.3%) and the Worcester area (South Worcestershire CCG) (16.8%).

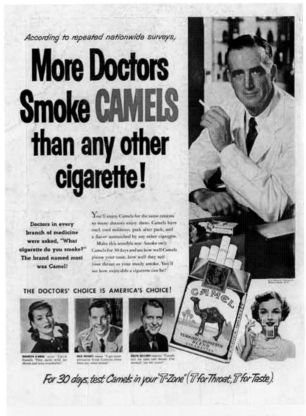

Figure 101 Cigarette smoking was heavily promoted as a healthy pastime throughout the US and UK until the late 20th century
(Martin Criminale, cc-by-sa/2.0,https://www.flickr.com/photos/itsnitram/8549712487/)

Smoking rates both in and outside of London are positively correlated with deprivation scores (index of multiple deprivation), with higher smoking rates found in areas of low social status. This is unlike in the past where the skeletal evidence indicated that pipe smoking was taken up by high and low status individuals alike. This represents a cultural change in attitudes towards smoking over time, leading to an overall reduction in smoking rates observed in the 20th century data. In 1974, 50% of men and 40% of women in the UK were smokers. This had fallen substantially to 19.1% and 14.9% respectively in 2015. James I would be pleased! However, air pollution is now considered to be the 'new tobacco' according to the World Health Organisation. Particulate air pollution today is a greater threat than smoking, shortening average global life expectancy by 1.8 years, making it 'the single greatest threat to human health'.

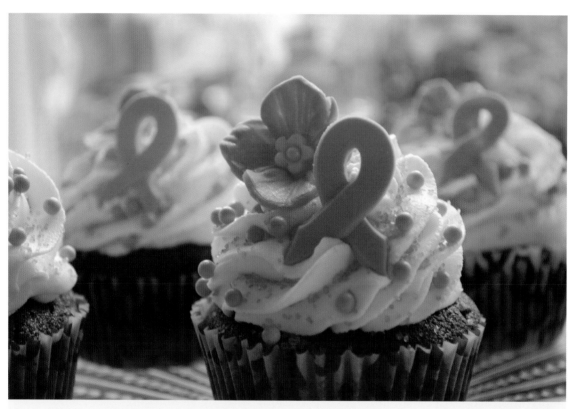
Figure 102 (Dixie Belle Cupcake Cafe, Texas, USA)

3

Cancer

Every 4 minutes someone in the UK dies from cancer (Cancer Research UK). It is an epidemic in modern Britain, with rates gradually increasing. Between 2014 and 2016, 164,000 deaths in the UK were caused by cancer, representing approximately 28% of all deaths. The most common cancers, those of the lung, bowel, breast and prostate, collectively comprised 45% of all cancer deaths. Cancer most frequently affects the older adult age group, with just over half of cancer deaths occurring in those over 75 years of age, though specific types of cancer affect people of different age groups. Cancer is currently the second most common cause of death in London and is the primary reason for premature death in the City (Cancer Commissioning Strategy for London).

Current scientific research suggests that lifestyle and environmental factors are involved in 90–95% of all cancers. Clinical data tells us that there is no single underlying cause of cancer and that there are, in fact, many risk factors leading to what is termed as 'preventable cancer'. These include, in order of number of cases per year in 2015 (Cancer Research UK):

- Tobacco (54,271)
- Obesity (22,761)
- UV radiation (13,604)
- Occupation (13,558)
- Infections (HPV, H. Pylori, EBV, HIV, Hepatitis, HTLV-1, liver worms and blood worms) (13,086)
- Alcohol (11,894)
- Insufficient fibre (11,693)
- Ionising radiation (6954)
- Processed meat (5352)

- Air pollution (3591)
- Not breastfeeding (2582)
- Insufficient physical activity (1917)
- Post-menopausal hormones (1371)
- Oral contraceptives (807)

Many of these risk factors are commonly seen as being symptomatic of our modern lifestyles, highly influenced by industrialisation and the technological revolution. So was cancer as prevalent in the UK before industrialisation? Have the resulting changes in our living environments and lifestyles triggered what we know today to be a disease on the increase? What do we really know about cancer in the past?

Detecting cancer in the past

Without modern technology, the earlier periods of medical history were entirely dependent upon empirical judgements and very limited observations made on externally visible signs and symptoms. We know that cancer was a recognised disease from the writings of Hippocrates (*c.* 460–370 BC), Celsus (*c.* 25 BC–AD 50) and Galen (AD 129–*c.* 210), documents which subsequently formed the basis of medical instruction for medieval physicians throughout Western Europe (Fig. 103), but *in vivo* only cancers affecting the outside of the body would have been identified, such as cancer of the mouth, scrotum or breast. Palpation (touch), however, could be a tool in identifying cancerous nodules and the enlargement of the spleen or liver.

Medical teaching during the medieval period maintained that cancer was incurable, although amputation of the affected part was recommended to prolong life. The term 'cancer' was quite widely applied to numerous conditions that today we know to be distinct conditions, such as penetrating abscesses, canker sores and shingles. It was a broadly used category of illness but at the same time also referred to the specific and malignant illness of 'morbid swellings' (apostemes), consisting of hard protrusions with dark veins like the legs of a crab (hence the coining of the name 'cancer') that spread quickly, eventually leading to ulcerous sores. By at least the 12th century in Western Europe, the development of distinctive cancerous growths was classified into detailed stages. It was believed that they were caused by corrupted, hardened or scorched black bile, one of the four humours of the body. Some cancers, including breast cancer, were also thought to have an undetectable, hidden phase, perhaps seated in the nerves or blood vessels.

With the granting of the charter for the creation of the *Company of Barber-Surgeons*

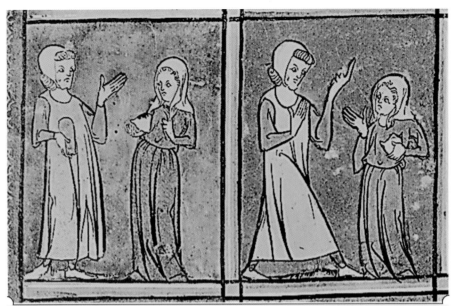

Figure 103 Medical breast examination. Extract from *Practica Rogerii*, an illuminated medical manuscript, 13th century

in London in 1540, Henry VIII also allowed, for the first time, the dissection of human cadavers. The Company could obtain the bodies of four executed criminals a year to expand their knowledge of human anatomy and pathology as well as practice surgical techniques. From this point onwards, medical knowledge grew rapidly, with London and its teaching hospitals forming the focus of medical learning within England. Many 'Barber Chyrurgeons' trained in London before returning to their home counties to work, rapidly spreading the latest medical developments out across the country, while most medical students from Oxford and Cambridge Universities also attended anatomy courses in London prior to returning to read for a degree in medicine. The first purpose-built medical school in the country was the Medical College at the London Hospital, which was founded in 1785, where students observed the practical skills of operating and undertaking amputations. The first hospital in the world specialising in cancer treatment was founded as the Free Cancer Hospital in Cannon Row, Westminster in 1851, which is now known as the Royal Marsden (Fig. 104). Cancer wards in smaller hospitals soon became common (Fig. 105).

Breast cancer became a dominant focus in oncology early on due to it presenting externally (Fig. 106). In fact, prior to the 20th century, this frequent identification of tumours in the breast and uterus led to cancer predominantly being framed as a 'woman's disease'. The observation by Walter Walshe in 1846, that a greater number

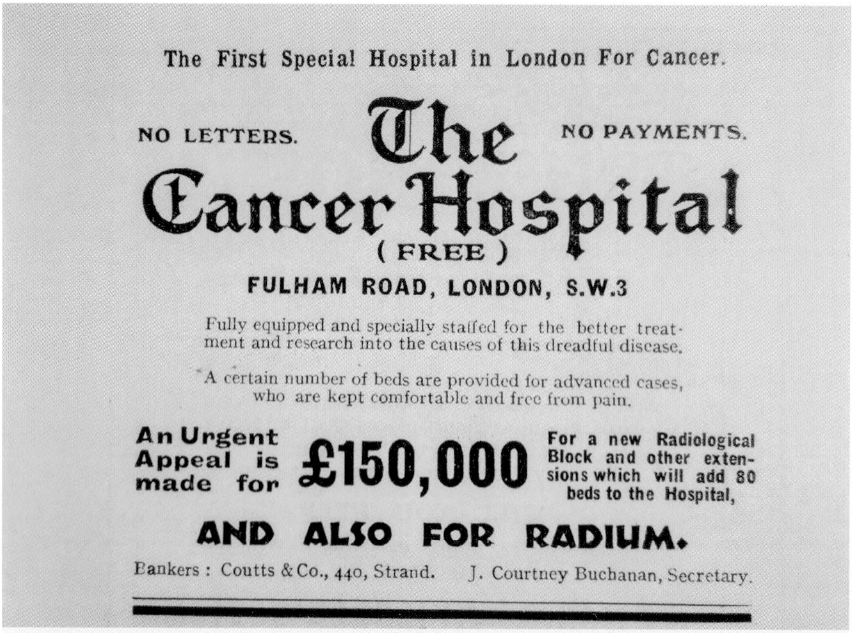

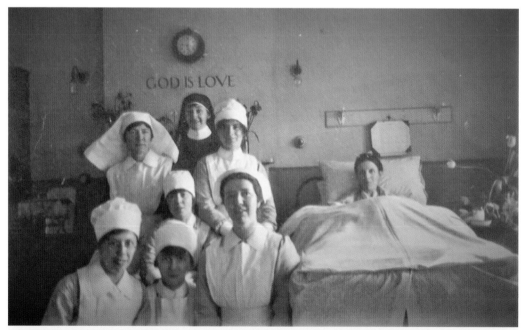

Figure 104 Advertisement from 1931 for appeal to raise funds for the Free Cancer Hospital (known today as the Royal Marsden)

(public domain)

Figure 105 Night and day staff of cancer ward, St Columba's Hospital, Hampstead, London, 1920s ('Tommy, Bunny, Lewis, Cooper, 'self', Sister Wright', patient in bed Miss Voogdt)

(public domain)

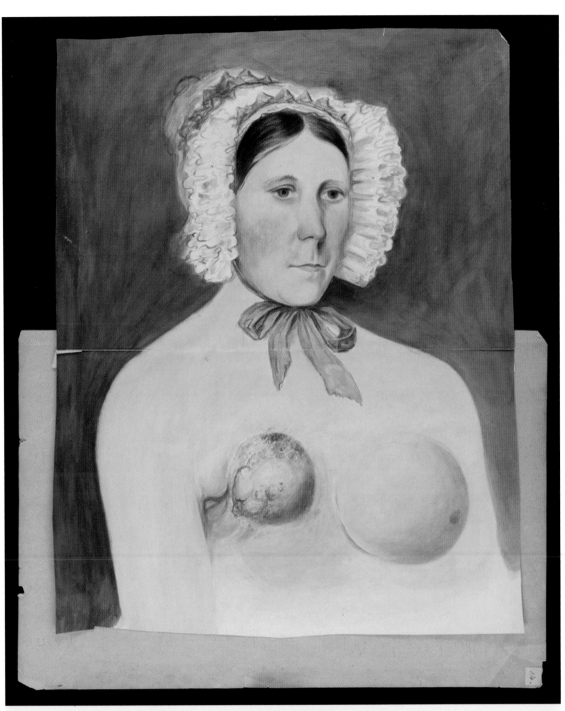

Figure 106 *Mrs Broadbent, Afflicted with Breast Cancer*, 1840, Watercolour

of females were reported to be affected by cancer, at 'a rate of two and three quarter times that of males', is not surprising. Examining mortality statistics from Paris, Walshe found that of the 9118 cancer related deaths, 2996 were classified as 'uterine' (cancer of the body of the uterus and the cervix uteri), 1147 as breast cancer and 64 as ovarian cancer. In comparison, only 21 cases of cancer of the testicles were reported along with only five cases of prostate cancer and five cases of male breast cancer. A similar finding is also reflected in the cancer mortality (death) statistics for 1851–1860 for the sites in our sample where, of all adult cancer deaths, on average 72.7% occurred in women compared to 27.3% in men (Fig. 107). However, by 1908, William Roger Williams reported that men were increasingly succumbing to these 'women's diseases' during the late 19th century due to their 'want of proper exercise and excess of food'. Not only that, at the turn of the 20th century, it was deemed that men were singularly subject to cancers of the lip and oral cavity of their own doing, since they were thought to be caused by irritation from the excessive use of unglazed pipe stems, alcohol consumption and poor oral hygiene.

Surgical intervention was still very limited in scope due to the lack of general anaesthesia in theatre until 1846, when diethyl ether and chloroform were first used for thoracic and abdominal procedures. Many operations carried out even after the invention of general anaesthesia were still not very successful due to post-

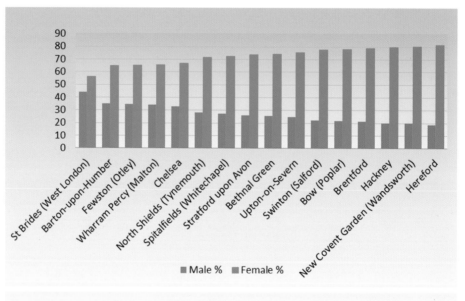

Figure 107 Cancer mortality as diagnosed according to sex in 1851–1860 (General Registrar's death records)

surgical (iatrogenic) infection. Nonetheless, some early cases of cancer diagnosis and subsequent surgical intervention are recorded. For example, in Stratford-upon-Avon, surgery for breast cancer was undertaken by the Clerk of Bridgnorth and Leach of Sturbridg (Shropshire) in the mid-17th century. The resection of the tumour appears to have been successful, at least in part. After the patient's death in 1666, Mr John Ward, rector of the Holy Trinity Church and medical practitioner along with a fellow medic, Mr Eedes, undertook a post-mortem examination to find that the tumour had regrown but had not spread to the ribs.

The fact that cancer could spread and involve multiple organs was well known very early on. For example, in 1320, Henri de Mondeville identified that the 'glands' were involved in cancer. LeDran (1685–1770), who recognised that some cancers could be cured if treated in the early stages, regularly removed enlarged axillary lymph nodes when undertaking mastectomies. Post-mortem examinations, undertaken at the behest of the Coroner and more routinely from the inception of the *Medical Witnessing Act* 1836, further confirmed the presence of tumours in organs that went undiagnosed during life. However, the mechanisms behind its spread were not known and were much speculated about. Cancer was likened to a poison and some thought it might be contagious. Others believed it to be a generalised disease that spread through 'cancer juices' as per the prevailing understanding of illnesses at the time to be an imbalance of the four bodily humours.

Only when fine lens microscopes were developed in the mid-19th century did the observations of medical researchers such as Schwann, in 1839, Walshe, in 1851, and Virchow, in 1859, lead to the development of 'cell theory' and 'cellular pathology'. In the 1860s, surgeons Charles Moore and William De Morgan of the Middlesex Hospital of London, which had a dedicated cancer ward from the late 18th century, espoused the belief that all cancers were the result of degenerative changes in the cells. By the meeting of the Pathological Society in London reported in 1874, the new cell theory was widely accepted. Not long after came the realisation that cells, being the basic biological unit of all living organisms, could not only be either healthy or pathological but that there could be a pathological multiplication of cells, or what is now called 'pathological cellular hyperplasia'; the modern clinical definition of cancer. As a result, it became evident that these superabundant pathological cells could spread to other parts of the body from a primary tumour through the lymph nodes and that this was one mechanism through which cancer in its later stages could affect multiple organs.

Today's cancer biology

The discovery of cells and cellular pathology that propelled cancer research onto a new level was then later augmented by a second major step in our knowledge of human biology: the creation of the first correct double helix model of DNA structure, as revealed through X-Ray diffraction in 1953 by Watson and Crick. Today's scientific research into cancer now focuses on both cellular structure and its controlling DNA.

Our current understanding is that cancer occurs when mutations take place in a progenitor cell's genome. Progenitor cells can be likened to a prototype about to develop into a specific type of cell. The genome of a progenitor cell, which consists of DNA, histones and other biochemical compounds that help package the DNA, controls its biochemical structure and its biochemical reactions. A healthy progenitor cell has a limited ability to replicate. However, if certain mutations occur in a progenitor cell's genome, it can develop the ability to continue to replicate perpetually, penetrate normal body surfaces and barriers (i.e. invade local tissues) and spread to other sites within the body (metastasize) via the lymphatic vessels and/or the blood vessels.

Multiple mutations of a cell's genome occurring over the lifetime of an individual are required for cancer to develop (Fig. 108). These mutations result from damage

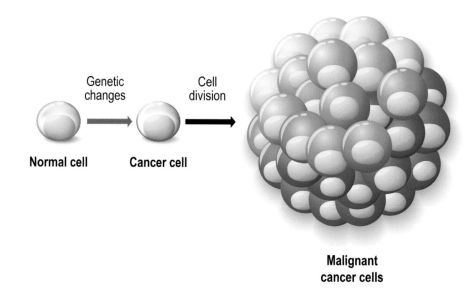

Genetic
changes

Cell
division

Normal cell   **Cancer cell**

**Malignant
cancer cells**

Figure 108 Mutation of a cell's genes leading to an abnormal cancer cell and its proliferation

(Shutterstock.com)

caused to the DNA by exogenous (environmental) or endogenous (metabolic) events and can also be inherited (5–10% of all cancers are suspected to develop due to a 'hereditary cancer syndrome', or an inherited increased lifetime risk of cancer).

A clear example of an exogenous factor is tobacco smoke, which is now known to contain genotoxic agents (mutagens) that damage the DNA of progenitor cells. Defective DNA repair of this damage subsequently leads to a mutation of the progenitor cell's genome. This results in its malfunction and a pathological proliferation of the mutated malignant cells, eventually causing lung cancer. The major exogenous carcinogenic mutagen in tobacco smoke is Benzo [alpha]pyrene, which is also found in urban air, chargrilled foods, vehicle exhaust fumes, asphalt and coke ovens (Fig. 109). It is highly likely that exogenous and endogenous factors interact and some mutagens can occur both exogenously and endogenously, so it can be difficult to quantify and differentiate between carcinogenic factors.

The most commonly mutated gene in all cancers is TP53 which, in its normal state, encodes a protein (p53) that suppresses tumours. If this protein is defective, cells can instead proliferate. Compromise of the TP53 gene may occur through inheriting only one functional copy of the gene or through damage incurred through exogenous mutagens such as viruses, chemicals or radiation. The tumour suppressor protein p53 can also be inactivated following infection with human papillomavirus (HPV).

Also of importance is the consequence of telomere length regulation. Telomeres are nucleoprotein

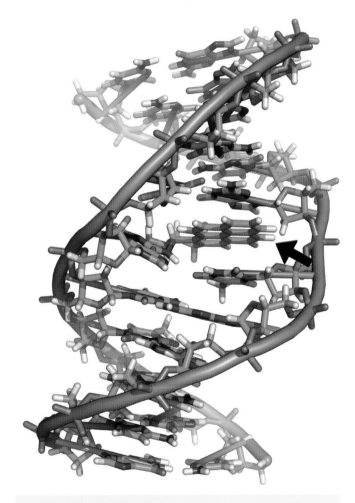

Figure 109 Segment of DNA bound to cancer causing chemical Benzo[alpha] pyrene (BaP), found in coal tar, tobacco smoke and foods, especially grilled meats

(Richard Wheeler, cc-by-sa/3.0, https://en.m.wikipedia.org/wiki/Benzo(a)pyrene)

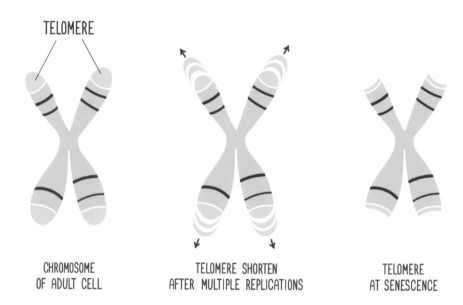

TELOMERE

CHROMOSOME
OF ADULT CELL

TELOMERE SHORTEN
AFTER MULTIPLE REPLICATIONS

TELOMERE
AT SENESCENCE

Figure 110 Telomeres that protect DNA in chromosomes shorten with age, exposing DNA to damage
(Shutterstock.com)

structured caps located at the ends of chromosomes that act to protect the end of the chromosomes to prevent DNA damage and also to protect genetic information during cell division.

As cells divide, telomeres shorten. Therefore, the natural progressive cell division that occurs in our bodies over the course of our lifetime as part of healthy regulatory maintenance leads to shorter and shorter telomeres as we age. Eventually, telomeres get too short to function and our cells begin to age (senescence) and die (apoptosis) (Fig. 110). Longer telomeres are therefore associated with continued cell proliferation and are now thought to increase risk for a number of cancers (Fig. 111).

According to one recent study, individuals with longer telomeres are a third more likely to develop any cancer than those with shorter telomeres. Risk varies according to the type of cancer, so that those with longer telomeres have a 66% higher risk of getting lung cancer, a 39% higher risk of breast cancer and a 55% higher risk of prostate cancer. The associations between telomere length and risk of cancer are not straightforward, however, and the complexities of this new area of research continue to be rapidly explored.

Despite the ground-breaking research currently being carried out into cancer, its causes and treatment, we still know very little about it in the past. The history of cancer before the modern clinical era is difficult to evaluate due to the restricted

Cancer development

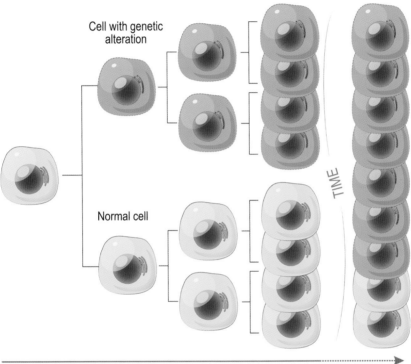

Cancerous cells do not submit to senescence or apoptosis. Continuous division of cells that take over healthy cells.

Cell with genetic alteration

Normal cell

TIME

Senescence is process, from the first cell division to apoptosis

Figure 111 Longer telomeres promote cell proliferation as we age
(Shutterstock.com)

nature of the early medical practitioners to observe, understand and diagnose the disease. The recognition and recording of cancer in patients have therefore varied widely over time, especially with regard to the biological sex of the individual, and it is unclear from historical documents as to whether prevalence rates of cancer have really increased substantially over human history. In order to provide an objective assessment of the presence of cancer in the past and whether it has increased in prevalence over time, we need to undertake diagnostic screening of human skeletal remains using the digital imaging technologies that are used to detect cancers today.

Metastatic bone disease

In using human skeletal remains as the focus for research into the presence of cancer in the past, by definition we are restricted to searching for evidence of cancers affecting the bone. This means that osteologists are very rarely able to be precise about the specific type of cancer present because we do not have the evidence from soft tissues. This affects our ability to compare prevalence rates of cancer in past populations with clinical data. Nonetheless, it is very common for the most frequent cancers to spread or metastasize from a primary tumour or generalised site to bone. Up to 85% of cancer patients have been found to have bone metastasis at autopsy. Metastatic bone disease is also the most common malignant cancer in the skeleton.

The cellular structure and composition of bone make it a highly targeted area for metastasizing cancer cells. Marrow stromal cells and bone matrix are able to attach themselves to adhesive molecules produced by cancerous tumours. Bone contains several growth factors (such as transforming growth factor β, insulin growth factors I and II, fibroblast growth factors, platelet derived growth factors and bone morphogenetic proteins), which can be released when tumour cells destroy bone. These growth factors act in synergy to promote further bone remodelling and further tissue factor release. Metastatic bone lesions are most frequently found in the skeletal elements that are high in red marrow content and where blood flow is high, i.e. the ribs, vertebrae, pelvis and hips that are supplied via Batson's venous plexus, a network of veins lacking valves that provides a route for metastases to spread (Fig. 112).

The most common cancers leading to bone metastases are known as the **BPLKT** cancers:

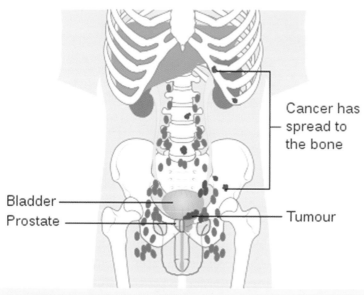

Cancer has spread to the bone

Bladder

Prostate

Tumour

Figure 112 Prostate cancer that has spread to the bone (blue areas), green dots representing lymph nodes

Breast
Prostate
Lung
Kidney
Thyroid

BPLKT tumours account for 80% of bone metastases (Table 12). Bone metastases can be either bone forming (osteoblastic), cause bone destruction (osteolysis) or can be a combination of both (mixed). Neither the type of metastatic bone lesion nor their distribution about the skeleton is absolutely indicative of the primary site of the cancer present. Nominal categories such as 'breast' and 'lung' cancer are umbrella terms covering several different types of specific cancers (i.e. adenocarcinoma, squamous cell carcinoma, large cell carcinoma), many of which are sub-classifications of the predominant BPLKT cancer, carcinoma. Carcinoma is a malignant type of cancer that develops from epithelial cells, one of the four basic types of animal tissue. In fact, approximately 90% of cancers arise in the simple epithelia that coat the internal organs.

There is a tendency for BPKLT cancers to produce particular types of metastatic bone lesions at different locations in the skeleton (Fig. 113). Overall, however, because of the overlap between these types and distributions, metastases are considered to be non-specific and diagnoses in human skeletal remains are more

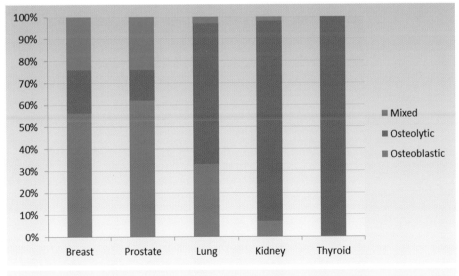

Figure 113 Types of bone metastases according to cancer type (after Justin Reddington, 2016)

Table 12 Facts about BPLKT cancers

(Cancer Research UK and Reddington 2016)

Type	Estimated % metastasize	Elements affected	Type of radiographic lesions	Ten year survival rate estimates	Risk factors	Prevalence 2003–2005/ *1993–1995	Prevalence 2013–2015
Breast Cancer	73%	Pelvis, vertebrae, femur, ribs, skull and humerus	Osteolytic 56% Osteoblastic 20% Mixed 24%	Females: 78%	Being overweight or obese • Alcohol • Contraceptive pill • Hormone replacement therapy • Being inactive • Age (rare in women under 40) • Family history and inherited genes • Height • Increased levels of sex hormones and insulin like growth factor 1 (IGF-1), which in turn is related to our genes, body weight and how much exercise we do • There is no evidence linking breast cancer risk to diet or smoking	Females: 134.8 per 100,000 Males: 1.4 per 100,000	Females: 170.0 per 100,000 Males: 1.4 per 100,000
Prostate Cancer	80%	Spine, ribs, pelvis, femur, sternum and skull	Osteoblastic 62% Mixed 24% Osteolytic 14%	84%	• Age (rare in those under 50) • Family history and genes • Being overweight or obese • Height • Insulin like growth factor (IGF-1) • Exposure to cadmium (in tobacco smoke, vegetables, meats, grains and fish)	114.7 per 100,000	172.6 per 100,000
Lung Cancer	33%	Rib, thoracic and lumbar vertebrae, pelvis and proximal femur	Osteolytic 64% Osteoblastic 33% Mixed 3%	5%	• Smoking tobacco (80% caused by smoking) • Exposure to radon gas (3%) (highest in the SW areas and builds up in homes and other buildings) • Chemicals and work-place risks (asbestos, silica, diesel engine exhaust fume exposure) • Air pollution • Family history • Lowered immunity	*Males from 140.9 per 100,000 *Females 52.6 per 100,000	Males 91.8 per 100,000 Females 67.9 per 100,000

Type	Estimated % metastasize	Elements affected	Type of radiographic lesions	Ten year survival rate estimates	Risk factors	Prevalence 2003–2005/ *1993–1995	Prevalence 2013–2015
Kidney Cancer	25%	Scapula, spine, pelvis and proximal femur	Osteolytic 91% Osteoblastic 7% Mixed 2%	50%	• Body weight • Height • Smoking • Kidney disease • Faulty genes and inherited conditions • Family history • High blood pressure • Alcohol • Thyroid cancer • Diabetes • Hysterectomy • Mild painkillers	*11.0 per 100,000 to	20.8 per 100,000
Thyroid Cancer	13%	Vertebrae (thoracic and lumbar), pelvis, ribs, skull and femur	Almost always Osteolytic	85%	• Being female • Advancing age • Family history • Radiation exposure • It is suspected that a combination of environmental factors, iodine deficiency and genetic factors (i.e. BRAF mutations) may explain the rising incidence of differentiated thyroid cancer, particularly more aggressive, late stage disease	*2.2 per 100,000	5.6 per 100,000

generally classified as metastatic bone disease or metastatic carcinoma. Clinically, in approximately 9% of metastatic bone disease cases, the location of the primary tumour is not identified.

Detecting cancer in human skeletal remains

Traditionally, human skeletal remains have been examined by osteologists using only the naked eye (macroscopically) with limited use of modern digital clinical imaging. Examples of cancers have been found but only in relatively small numbers compared to other diseases regularly observed in archaeological assemblages. To date, it has been unclear as to whether more cases of metastatic bone disease would be found if modern digital imaging such as radiography and CT scanning were used to analyse the internal structure of skeletal elements, rather than being restricted to examining only the outside of the bone macroscopically. It could be the case that metastatic bone lesions occurring within the bone structure without penetrating the bone surface remain undetected.

We undertook a digital radiographic survey of a total of 2241 individuals from archaeological assemblages (Figs 114 and 115) in order to identify evidence for cases of metastatic bone disease in past populations using diagnostic clinical criteria. Individuals from London and outside of the City were included, from both the Industrial and pre-Industrial periods.

Our survey included the key skeletal elements affected by metastatic bone disease: lumbar vertebrae, pelvis (os coxae), femur (left) and cranium (Fig. 116). Radiography was only undertaken on skeletal elements in good condition, with a note being made of any post-mortem damage present which might be mistaken for metastatic lesions (pseudolesions). Radiographs were also compared to the photographic images or the elements themselves where possible to aid the correct identification of post-mortem damage.

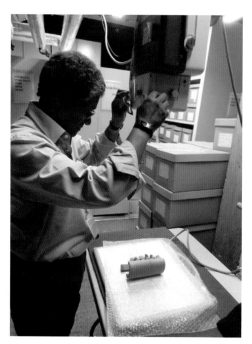

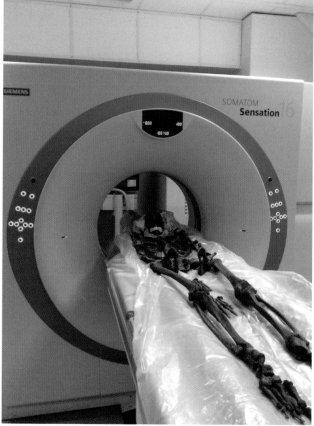

Figure 114 (left) Wayne Hoban (Reveal Imaging Ltd) undertaking radiographic imaging
(J. Bekvalac)

Figure 115 (right) CT scanning human skeletal remains
(J. Bekvalac)

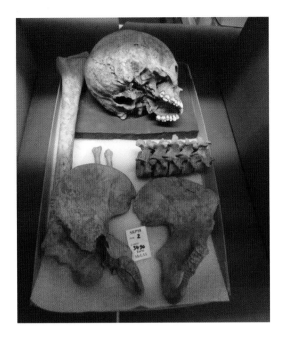

Digital radiography is a rapid method of imaging the internal bone structure, with previews of the radiographic images provided instantly (Fig. 117). Where pathological changes were observed at the time of the radiography, extra elements could then also be examined. In a clinical context, radiography is not as sensitive to bone changes as other imaging modalities such as MRI and CT scanning, however, because at least 40% of bone density must be lost before any changes are evident. Although some elements were also examined using CT scanning to compare to our radiographic observations, it is still possible, as is the case in the clinical setting, that some metastatic lesions would not have been observed.

A

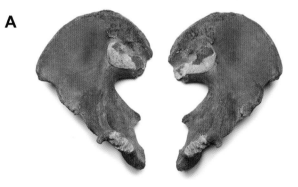

B

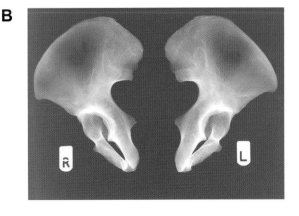

Metastatic bone disease data comparison

To examine rates of metastatic bone disease (MBD) over time, analysis of prevalence rates are based on populations of deceased persons (past populations) rather than in reference to the living population. The age demographic of past populations needs to be taken into account as cancer occurs most commonly in older individuals. Since BPLKT cancers tend to appear from middle age onwards (35 years and upwards), calculations here are based on the combined total of middle aged and old aged individuals. This also helps circumvent issues identifying old age individuals in archaeological populations, where age estimates for adults are broad. Where a specific age at death is known from biographical records, this was used to categorise the age of an individual.

In the UK in 2016, 5.78% of the total number of middle aged and old aged adult males and 2.46% of the total number of the middle aged and old aged adult females who died are estimated to have had BPLKT metastases. This estimate is based on the average number of annual BPLKT cancer deaths in 2014–2016 (Cancer Research UK), the percentage of those cancers expected to metastasize and the total number of middle aged (35–49 years) and old aged (50+ years) deaths amongst males and females in the UK in 2016 (Office of National Statistics). An estimate of 4.08% of all middle aged and old aged adult individuals who died in 2016 are likely to have had BPLKT metastases.

Given that BPLKT cancers are the origin of approximately 80% of all bone metastases, rates of metastatic bone disease from BPLKT cancers should be considered as a minimum of the total metastatic bone disease present. Estimates for all cancer bone metastases may be around 5.10%, with approximately 7.23% of middle aged and old aged males who died in 2016 and approximately 3.08% of middle aged and old aged females who died in 2016 having had metastatic bone disease (assuming an average of *c*. 44% metastatic rate, the average rate for BPLKT bone metastasis).

Our radiographic analysis of archaeological human skeletal remains identified five definite cases of metastatic bone disease amongst a total number of 573 middle aged and old aged females (0.87%; Table 13). Two further cases were found in the 798 middle aged and old aged males examined (0.25%; Figs 118 and 119). The total prevalence rate of metastatic cases in the middle aged and old aged sample was 0.51% (N=1371). The prevalence rates of metastatic bone disease increased over time (Fig. 120). More cases were found in the total Industrial period London population (0.71%) than in either the pre-Industrial London sample (0%) or in either industrial (0.21%) or pre-Industrial populations outside of London (0.36%). Only half of the cases identified radiographically had previously been identified macroscopically.

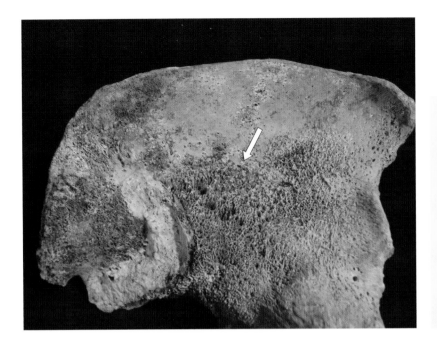

Figure 118 (left)
Left pelvis of old adult male, Industrial London (SB79 102) with osteoblastic metastatic bone disease

(J. Bekvalac)

Figure 119 (below)
Digital radiograph of pelves and sacrum with mottled appearance from mixed lesions of lucency and increased density, indicative of metastatic bone changes, old adult male, Industrial London (SB79 102)

(© Museum of London)

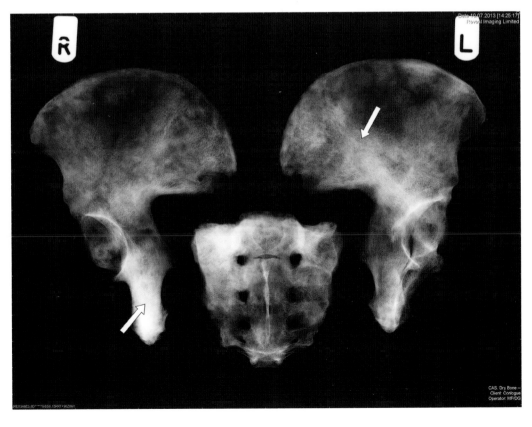

Table 13 Prevalence rates of metastatic bone disease (MBD) according to age and population in female (F) and male (M) Adults, according to age (YA = young adult, MA = middle adult and OA = old adult)

	FYA	FMA	FOA	MYA	MMA	MOA	Total
MBD cases	1	2	1	0	1	1	6
Industrial London	153	106	186	94	109	194	842
%	0.65	1.89	0.54	0	0.92	0.52	0.71
MBD cases	0	0	1	0	0	0	1
Industrial non-metropolitan	96	58	39	82	104	97	476
%	0	0	2.56	0	0	0	0.21
MBD cases	0	0	0	0	0	0	0
Pre-Industrial London	125	62	31	131	113	47	509
%	0	0	0	0	0	0	0
MBD cases	0	1	0	0	0	0	1
Pre-Industrial non-metropolitan	89	55	36	100	70	64	414
%	0	1.8	0	0	0	0	0.24
MBD cases	1	3	2	0	1	1	8
Total	463	281	292	407	396	402	2241
%	0.22	1.07	0.68	0	0.25	0.25	0.36

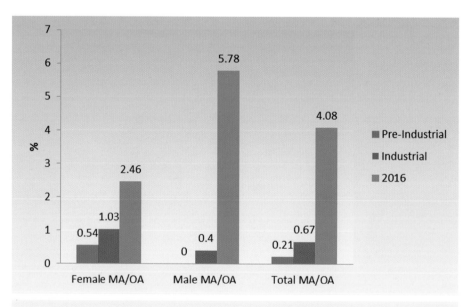

Figure 120 Metastatic bone disease prevalence rates by period in male and female middle aged (MA) and old aged (OA) adults (2016 based on BPLKT metastatic prevalence rates)

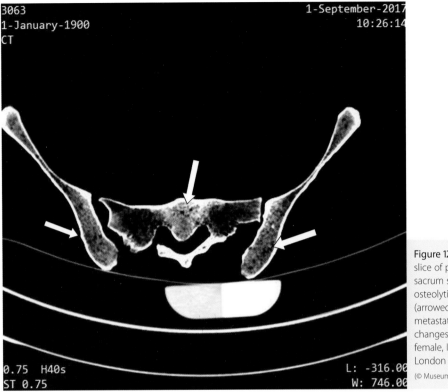

Figure 121 CT scan slice of pelves and sacrum showing osteolytic lesions (arrowed) indicating metastatic bone changes, middle adult female, Industrial London (PGV10 3063)

Within the archaeological industrial sample, eight females of known identity also had a record of the cause of death noted at the time either on death certificates or in burial records. Only two of these (25%) had diagnostic MBD changes that could be detected radiographically (Fig. 120). This discrepancy could be due to a number of factors: the cause of death could have been misdiagnosed; the particular cancers present (not detailed) may not have led to metastatic bone disease or may have led to MBD in skeletal elements not examined here; or some individuals in the past with malignant cancers did not survive long enough to develop MBD.

Multiple myeloma

Multiple myeloma (MM) is a cancer of plasma cells that results in bone lesions (Fig. 122) that can also be detected using radiography. Plasma cells are white blood cells that originate from B lymphocyte cells in bone marrow and normally secrete antibodies. Damage occurring to the DNA of a plasma cell, caused by foreign substances during its development in the lymph or spleen, can result in the immune system's ability to

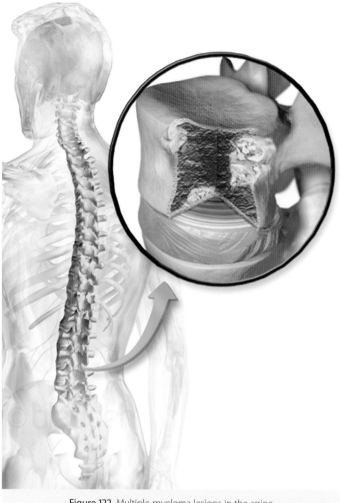

Figure 122 Multiple myeloma lesions in the spine
(Blausen Medical Communications, Inc. cc-by/3.0)

maintain normal levels of plasma cells and antibodies being compromised. This translocation or mutation results in the production of a damaged plasma cell clone that in turn leads to the proliferation of abnormal plasma cells in the bone marrow and the presence of an antibody, known as paraprotein, in the body. This condition is known as monoclonal gammopathy of undetermined significance (MGUS) but is a common, age-related condition that is often be asymptomatic. A further more advanced type of myeloma that is still asymptomatic is known as smouldering or indolent myeloma. This is a premalignant form of myeloma.

Over time, a series of such further genetic and epigenetic mutations of the abnormal plasma cells caused by foreign substances arising from the environment can lead to the production of more aggressive damaged plasma cell clones, eventually leading to higher levels of paraprotein and abnormal bone marrow plasma cells (myeloma cells), uncontrolled by the immune system. Most frequently in multiple myeloma cases, a chromosomal translocation between locus q32 on chromosome 14 and an oncogene (a gene with the potential not only to cause cancer by preventing the death of a malfunctioning cell but also to allow it to survive and proliferate) occurs. At this stage, the common symptoms of multiple myeloma may occur, including bone lesions, at which stage it is considered malignant. Myeloma cells accumulate in the bone marrow, forming tumours, and bone marrow stromal cells are stimulated to overproduce the RANKL protein that activates osteoclasts,

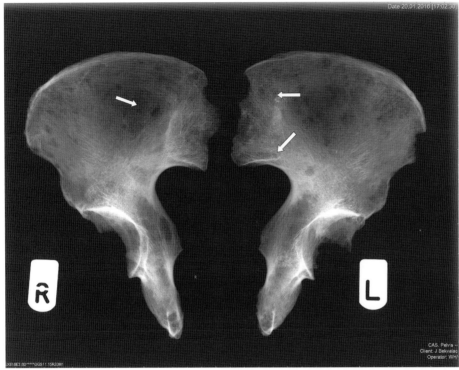

Figure 123 Digital radiograph of pelves with radiolucent rounded lesions (arrowed) diagnostic of multiple myeloma, old adult female, Industrial London (FAO90 1360)

(© Museum of London)

bone cells that resorb bone. This leads to diagnostic lesions in the skeleton that are clearly seen on radiographic images as radiolucent rounded or 'raindrop' lesions, appearing as holes (Fig. 123). The most commonly affected skeletal elements are the spine, skull, pelvis, ribs and long bones. Bone lesions occur in almost all cases of MM (Fig. 124).

No single cause of myeloma has been identified. Risk factors include having the MGUS condition, which precedes the development of almost all cases of multiple

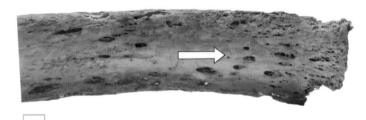

A

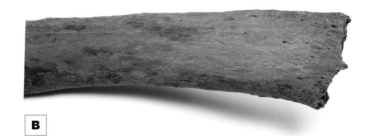

B

Figure 124 Sternal ends of ribs (visceral surface) (A) showing multiple lytic (destructive) bone lesions (arrow) indicating multiple myeloma, middle adult male, Industrial London (FAO90 1879); (B) rib with no pathological changes, middle adult male, Industrial London (PGV10 2588)

(© Museum of London)

myeloma, though only 1–2% of people a year with MGUS will develop MM. Similarly, smouldering myeloma carries an increased risk of developing MM, with 10% of cases developing into MM each year for the first 5 years. Obesity has also been identified as increasing an individual's risk of MM: an 11% increase in risk occurs at each increase by 5 of the body mass index. Other factors include age, being male, being of African descent, alcohol, radiation exposure, family history, autoimmune conditions, HIV, and chemicals such as ethylene oxide and benzene. Benzene is well known to cause bone marrow diseases and is now strictly regulated, especially in the work-place, but formerly was used in the 19th and 20th centuries as an after-shave lotion due to its sweet odour as well as to decaffeinate coffee as part of a new method invented in 1903 For the most part, benzene was extracted from coal tar and petroleum to be used as part of industrial processes from 1845 until the mid–late 20th century. Commercial production of ethylene oxide dates to the early 20th century and continues today as one of the most important raw materials for use in the production of plastics, polyester, antifreeze, perfumes and cosmetics. Ethylene oxide is a proven carcinogen and chronic exposure can result in the mutation of DNA.

The first recorded historical case of multiple myeloma was noted by Samuel Solly of Guy's Hospital, London in 1844 in a 39-year-old patient. In the UK, the earliest archaeological case in the published literature is a female dating to the late Roman period from Poundbury, Dorset, aged 35+ years at death.

Multiple myeloma data comparison
The average number of deaths from multiple myeloma in 2014–2016 in the UK per year in old age and middle age individuals was 2994 (0.51%, N=585,396), 1644 of which were in males (0.58%, N=285,552) and 1350 were in females (0.45%, N=299,844) (Cancer Research UK, Office of National Statistics).

In our radiographic survey of the industrial and pre-Industrial populations, four cases of multiple myeloma were found in the total middle aged and old aged sample, giving an overall prevalence rate of 0.29% (N=1371). Two cases were in old aged and middle aged adult females (0.35%, N=573) and two cases were in old aged adult males (0.25%, N=798). All the cases were from the industrial London sample (0.67%, N=595) with no cases found in any of our populations from pre-Industrial London or from outside of London. None of the cases had been diagnosed macroscopically.

According to our observations, rates of multiple myeloma have increased over time, with rates of MM almost doubling since the Industrial period, although it is still a relatively rare disease (Fig. 125). More recently, MM mortality rates are reported to have increased since the 1970s by 60% in the UK (Cancer Research UK).

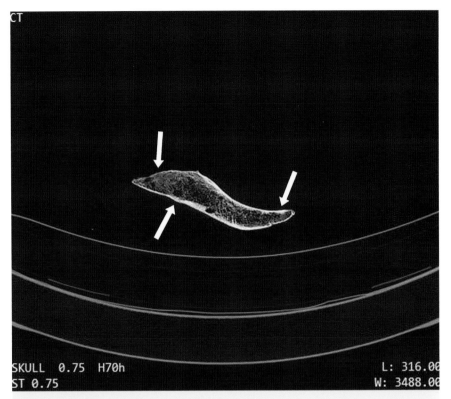

Figure 125 CT scan slice of left pelvis with multiple lytic lesions indicative of multiple myeloma, old adult female, Industrial London (FAO90 1360)

(© Museum of London)

Local trends in cancer

Although our archaeological sample is small compared to the size of modern populations, the radiographic data suggest that, in the past, London had higher rates of metastatic bone disease and multiple myeloma than areas outside of London and that these diseases were more common in the Industrial period than in the pre-Industrial era. Whilst we know from both archaeological cases and historic records that cancer has existed in humans throughout our history, our data indicates that the urbanisation of London and the industrial developments of its later history appear to have created human living environments and lifestyles that have accelerated rates of metastatic bone disease and multiple myeloma in both male and female adults. This appears to be part of an ongoing trend today.

Comparison of today's mortality statistics from our sites across the country indicate that cancer mortality rates differ according to locality (Fig. 126). London

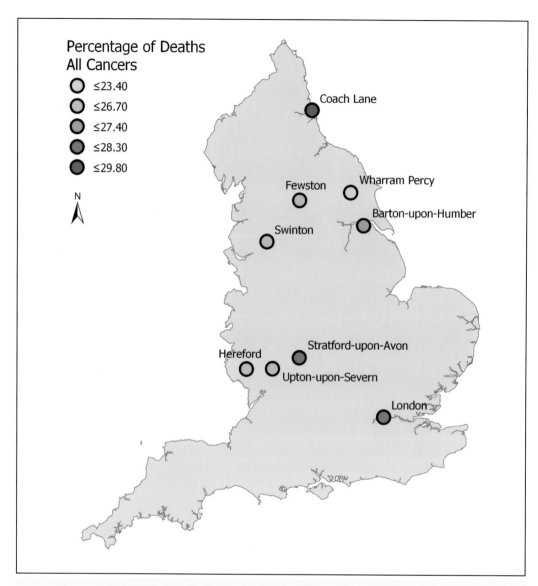

Figure 126 National Statistics for Cancer percentage mortality rates
(Cancer Research UK, 2013–2015, http://www.cancerresearchuk.org/health-professional/cancer-statistics/incidence)

(average 28.3%) and North Shields (North Tyneside CCG) (29.8%) have the highest percentage rates of cancer deaths compared to the lowest rates at Wharram Percy, East Yorkshire (Scarborough and Ryedale CCG) (23.4%) and at Fewston, North Yorkshire (Airedale, Wharfedale and Craven CCG) (26.4%). Variation in these mortality trends may relate to the local environments and lifestyles influencing cancer risk factors but these trends will also differ according to the local provision and take up

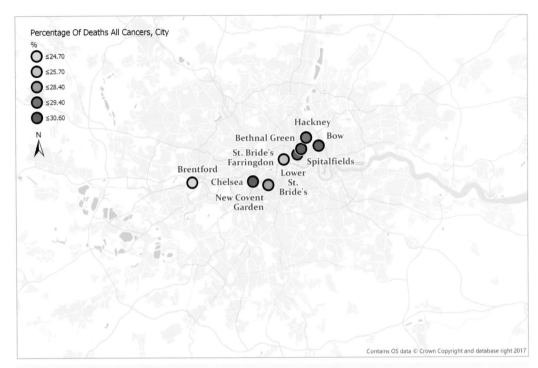

Figure 127 London statistics for Cancer percentage mortality rates

(Cancer Research UK, 2013–2015, http://www.cancerresearchuk.org/health-professional/cancer-statistics/incidence)

of medical screening, treatments and follow up care, increasing survival. For example, in contrast to mortality rates, the average prevalence rate of cancer in the living population in 2013–2015 across our sites in London was actually considerably lower (1.6 per 100,000) than that of our sites outside of London (average 3.1 per 100,000) (Fig. 127). Prevalence rates in living populations to at least some extent reflect early detection levels of cancer and the survival of cancer patients, rather than the total number of cases in local populations actually being higher or lower. As in the past, the way in which cancers are detected can influence the statistics reported: undetected cases will not be included.

In our sample, rates of cancer mortality within London today is strongly related to population density; less densely populous areas have lower cancer mortality rates than those that are more densely populated (Table 14). London not only has a higher than average rate of cancer diagnoses being made in A&E departments, rather than at earlier stages through routine screening, but also nine out of the ten worst hospitals for cancer care as reported by patients are in London (Cancer Commissioning Strategy for London). Population density puts health care under extreme pressure

Table 14 Population density London Boroughs, 2016 and cancer mortality percentage rates (Public Health England, 2013–2015)

	Density per km² 2016	Cancer mortality % all deaths
Hounslow	4843	24.7
Central London	3241	25.7
Wandsworth	9226	28.4
City and Hackney	14358	29.4
Tower Hamlets	15404	30.1
West London	12931	30.6

from not only the sheer numbers of people requiring services but also the complexities of organising and developing health service amenities within the congested metropolitan environment.

Several areas, both in and outside London, with high cancer mortality rates also have high levels of socioeconomic deprivation. Socioeconomic deprivation not only is often associated with lower uptake of cancer screening programmes but also with many lifestyle factors that put people at higher risk of developing cancer, such as smoking, being physically inactive, poor diet and obesity.

Rates of mortality from specific types of cancer will also vary irrespective of general cancer rates according to these factors. For example, age standardised lung cancer mortality rates per 100,000 in 2013–2105 were lower in Chelsea and Kensington (88.1) than in Tower Hamlets (117.7), as was excess weight in adults (47.3 compared to 52.5) and smoking rates (18.9 compared to 21.1). Overall, however, Chelsea and Kensington had a similar total percentage of cancer deaths for the same period (30.6%) as Tower Hamlets (30.1%). Both Tower Hamlets and Chelsea and Kensington have lower lung cancer mortality rates than Salford (128.0), which has not only the highest rate of lung cancer mortality in our group but also the highest rate of smoking (23.0) and the second highest rate of obesity (67.1). Overall, however, Salford had a lower rate of cancer deaths percentage rate (25.9%) than either Chelsea and Kensington or Tower Hamlets. For lung cancer, research suggests that socioeconomic status is the key factor in its prevalence and that when this is taken into account there is little difference between prevalence rates in rural and urban areas in England.

In the past, survival rates of cancer would have been very low. Thanks to our expanding epidemiological knowledge and research into its pathogenesis, cancer mortality rates in the UK are falling, and in fact have fallen by about 15% over the past 10 years, despite a continuing increase in prevalence. Overall, mortality rates in modern populations inform us about the impact of our local living environment on responses to disease incidence and on how amenities and education are developed to cope with our health needs as dictated by local circumstances. Population density, local variation in lifestyle factors as well as health service funding and delivery all have significant impacts on cancer outcomes. A European wide study found that in relation to all cancers, health expenditure per capita had a significant inverse relationship with mortality and a significant positive relationship with incidence in the living population (Université Libre de Bruxelles). In other words, the increased funding of health services results in lower cancer mortality rates and, subsequently, an increase in cancer incidence due to higher rates of early detection and survival. Today, cancer incidence and mortality are highly influenced both by the wealth of the countries and organisations funding cancer health care services and also by socioeconomic deprivation of areas at risk of cancer through associated lifestyle factors.

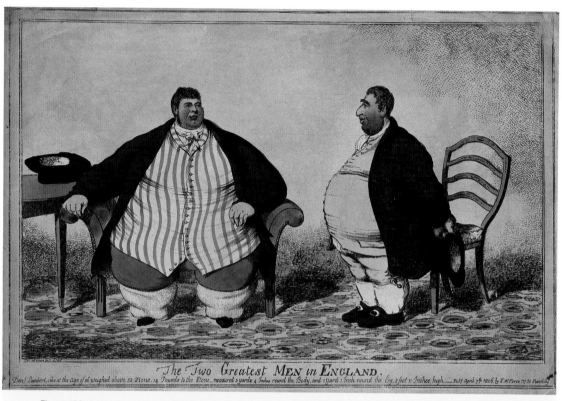

The Two Greatest MEN in ENGLAND.

Dan.ᵉˡ Lambert, who at the Age of 36 weighed above 50 Stone, 14 Pounds to the Stone, measured 3 yards 4 Inches round the Body, and 1 Yard 1 Inch round his Leg, 5 feet 11 Inches high. ___ Pub.ᵈ April 7.ᵗʰ 1806 by S.W. Fores 50 to Piccadilly.

Figure 128 *A Humorous Comparison Between the Obese Daniel Lambert and Charles James Fox*, 1806, coloured etching

4

Getting fat: a growing crisis

Britain is the fattest nation in Western Europe, according to the Organisation for Economic Co-operation and Development. In 2015, 62.9% of adults in the UK aged 15–74 years were either obese or overweight, affecting 58% of women and 68% of men. Obesity not only leads to serious and chronic health issues, including heart disease, cancer, diabetes, osteoarthritis, decreased lung function and shorter life expectancy, but, by 2030, it is estimated that the extra 11 million more obese people in the UK will result in health care costs of £1.9–2 billion a year. It's a big problem. But how long has it been going on and why is being fat so bad for us?

The problem with fat: cancer

Being obese puts the body into a chronic state of low grade inflammation. Traditionally, fat was viewed as just a reservoir for energy, with fat being generated as we eat more calories than we expend through exercise. Now, however, the latest science tells us that fat is actually a large gland – in fact, fat is the body's largest endocrine organ. In this capacity, fat is able to interact with other body systems to help maintain and regulate its metabolism and immunity. It can switch biological functions on or off. As an organ, adipose tissue (fat) is a finely balanced mechanism keeping anti-inflammatory and pro-inflammatory factors (cytokines) in check with immune cells. This allows healthy functioning of the endocrine system and systemic insulin action, contributing to normal whole body metabolism. If we get too fat, we break the system. This is particularly true if we gain abdominal fat, the result of adipose tissue expansion in the abdominal region. Adipocytes (specialist cells that store fat) increase in size and some start to collapse and die (apoptosis), a process known as adipocyte dysfunction. Prompted by the death of fat cells, macrophages arrive at the site to digest the dead cells as part of our natural system of immunity, a reaction called inflammation. The more fat there is, the more adipocytes there are going into apoptosis and the more macrophages there are in the fat tissue. In obese fat tissue, up to 40% of total cells present may be macrophages. Therefore, in obesity, fat is in a state of chronic inflammation.

The effect of this chronic inflammation is negative on the body because adipocyte dysfunction leads to the over-production of several cytokines (regulators of host response to infection) that are proinflammatory, including leptin, which plays a primary role in the proinflammatory process and may lead to cell proliferation. There are higher levels of leptin in obese people. Inflammation is a key factor in the development and progression of cancer. Numerous inflammatory cells and mediators are found in tumour microenvironments, where they can activate the proliferation and metastasis of cancer cells as well as the formation of new blood vessels (angiogenesis). Recent clinical research has identified that cells other than cancer cells present in tumour microenvironments play a key role in cancer pathogenesis. These include inflammatory and immune cells, cytokines and adipocytes. Chronic inflammation of adipose tissue therefore has a substantial effect on the tumour microenvironment with the result that excess fat directly contributes towards cancer progression.

Diabetes

Excess fat also leads to dysregulation of the metabolic system, affecting growth hormones such as insulin, as well as sex hormones testosterone and oestrogen. Insulin plays a vital role in the body's metabolism and controls how glucose is absorbed and processed. However, the body prioritises the use of free fatty acids from body fat over the use of glucose for energy. Cells then become increasingly resistant and desensitised to insulin and cannot take up glucose properly, so that glucose levels then increase in the blood. This is known as insulin resistance. In order to compensate for this and reduce blood glucose levels, the pancreas generates more insulin (hyperinsulinemia). Insulin resistance therefore leads to chronically raised levels of insulin. Higher levels of insulin have an impact on levels of growth factors (including insulin-like growth factor, IGF-1) available to cells, potentially leading to their proliferation. In response to both insulin and insulin-related growth

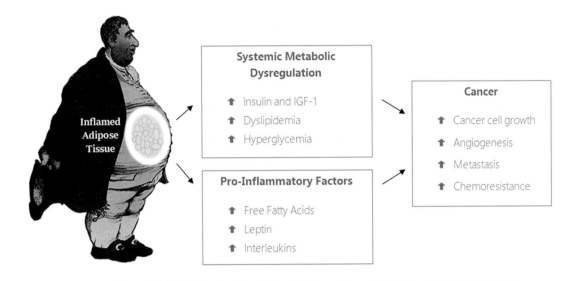

Figure 129 Relationships between fat, inflammation, hormones and cancer (after Tuo Deng *et al.* 2016)

factors, cancer cells are more resilient and also reproduce faster. Not only does the dysregulation of the metabolic system caused by being overweight or obese create states of insulin resistance, but the dysregulation of insulin caused by the simultaneous inflammation can also result in a significant increase in cancer risk because of the associated production of growth factors (Fig. 129).

Recent research has demonstrated that fat accumulating in the liver plays a vital role in the maintenance of the insulin regulation system, growth factors and sex hormones. A cycle occurs whereby hyperinsulinemia causes fatty liver, which then leads to increased insulin resistance, which in turn leads to increased hyperinsulinemia. As such, visceral fat (fat found in the abdominal cavity close to the vital organs) is a greater risk factor and therefore a more accurate predictor of diabetes compared to overall body weight.

Hormones

Insulin dysregulation caused by fatty liver can lead to increased levels of insulin, growth hormone, IGF-1 and androgens (male hormones). Obesity also leads to reductions in sex hormone-binding globule (SHBG), a protein that binds to the sex hormones oestrogen and testosterone, through sugar or monosaccharide induced hepatic lipogenesis (fat production in the liver) and changes in proinflammatory cytokines (TNF-alpha, interleukins (ILs) and adiponectin). There are complex interactions between SHBG and the sex hormones but, in essence, the binding of oestrogen and androgen to SHBG protects individuals from excessive quantities of either hormone; once bound to SHBG, oestrogen and testosterone are no longer 'bioavailable'. Reduction in the production of SHBG, therefore, generates higher levels of free testosterone and oestrogen, which can have a negative effect on health.

This is exacerbated in post-menopausal females who are overweight or obese since abdominal fat is a major source of testosterone and oestrogen in this age group. After the menopause, the ovaries no longer produce oestrogen and produce only 50% of testosterone. The remaining 50% of testosterone is produced in the peripheral tissues including body fat. Increased fat levels will therefore result in increased testosterone as well as reduced SHGB levels, leading to a marked increase of bioavailable oestrogen and testosterone in post-menopausal overweight or obese females. The biosynthetic conversion of pre-androgens (biochemical precursor to male hormones) and testosterone in fat tissue is the source of oestrogen. Oestrogen made by fat cells leads to the division of certain cells, such as mammary epithelial cells and intestinal stem cells, which are involved in cancer. Too much fat, therefore, leads to the proliferation of these cells due to the associated rise in oestrogen. There is a direct relationship between obesity, high oestrogen levels and breast and womb cancers. Oestrogen is also linked to higher rates of breast cancer in men and to higher rates of aggressive prostate cancer but it is not currently known if this is due to oestrogen or to testosterone, given the inter-relationship between the two hormones. The balance of the sex hormones corresponds to the biological sex of an individual, so dysregulation of the hormones can affect males and females in an inverse manner. For example, high testosterone levels in females are associated with insulin resistance, glucose intolerance and increased risk of type 2 diabetes. In males, high testosterone levels appear to perform the opposite function of helping to prevent insulin resistance and type 2 diabetes. Oestrogen, on the other hand, is associated with raised insulin levels in both sexes. Low SHBG plasma levels are similarly consistent in their association with insulin resistance and increased risk of type 2 diabetes in both sexes.

Metabolic syndrome

The cascade of biomolecular interactions we have seen stemming from obesity and, in particular, excess visceral fat, can lead to a cluster of conditions collectively known as metabolic syndrome or MetS. The co-occurring conditions that comprise metabolic syndrome are excess body fat around the waist, high blood sugar, increased blood pressure and abnormal cholesterol or triglyceride levels. An individual with at least three of these conditions is considered to have metabolic syndrome. Metabolic syndrome is a risk factor for other diseases, such as type 2 diabetes, cardiovascular disease, stroke, cirrhosis of the liver, dementia and polycystic ovarian syndrome. Causes are thought to include obesity, stress, genetics, ageing, sedentary lifestyle, low physical activity, disrupted sleep, mood disorders and excessive alcohol use. Prevalence of the condition increases significantly with age, reportedly rising from 11.0% in 20–29-year-old to 47.2% in 80–89-year-old males and from 9.2% to 64.4% in the same age groups for females. Post-menopausal women are at greater risk since the transition from the pre- to post-menopause involves the same factors involved in metabolic syndrome in tandem with a decrease in oestrogen. One of the key causes identified for metabolic syndrome is diet, in particular Western dietary habits heavily based on processed food and sugar-sweetened drinks.

Evidence for metabolic syndrome in the past: DISH

Two conditions that may be linked to metabolic syndrome that we see in human skeletal remains are Diffuse Idiopathic Skeletal Hyperostosis (DISH) and Hyperostosis Frontalis Interna (HFI). Both are conditions that result in extra bone being formed in the skeleton that are predominantly found in older aged adults. In DISH, the bone formation is seen in the spine and joints, with the characteristic pathognomic (diagnostic) changes present in the thoracic vertebrae. Here, the soft tissue spinal ligaments undergo ossification creating a bony bridge between the vertebrae. The bridge consists of a thick, dripping-wax like solid bone on the right hand side of the mid- and lower spine (Fig. 130). When four individual vertebrae are fused together by the bony bridge, DISH is diagnosed. Similar ossification of smaller ligaments about the spine and other extra-spinal soft tissue ligaments and tendons at the long bone joints and skeletal protuberances can also occur. DISH is usually seen clearly both macroscopically and radiographically.

The exact aetiology of DISH is not known and until recently has received little

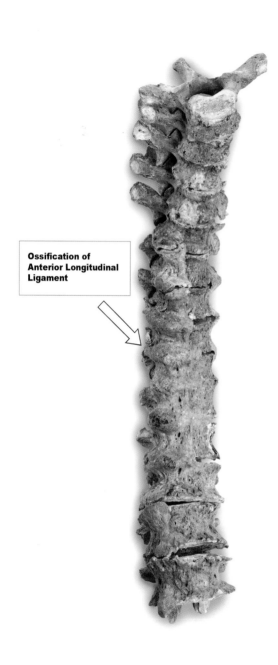

Ossification of Anterior Longitudinal Ligament

Figure 130 Vertebrae with 'wax like' bony fusion indicative of Diffuse Idiopathic Skeletal Hyperostosis (DISH) older male, Chelsea Old Church, Industrial London

(© Museum of London)

attention in the medical literature since, despite the dramatic skeletal changes, it is of little clinical significance other than producing a degree of stiffness in the spine. However, a handful of studies have brought some information to light. DISH and obesity are commonly associated, particularly in adults over 60 years old. Prevalence rates increased with age. The relationship between DISH and body mass index (BMI) as well as waist circumference has also been noted for both males and females, though DISH is most frequently found in males. DISH is also associated with hyperglycaemia or type 2 diabetes. One study found an increase of DISH from a rate of 4% in non-diabetic 60–69-year-old patients to 21% in the same age group who were diabetic. Overall prevalence rates of DISH have been found to be 17% in those over 50 years old, with rates of 22.7% in males compared to 12.1% of females. Interestingly, archaeological research undertaken on skeletal remains with DISH has made complementary discoveries, where dietary analysis has shown that individuals with DISH tend to have had enriched diets that were higher in meat or fish content.

It is thought that the metabolic factors (insulin, growth hormone and IGF-1) associated with hyperinsulinaemia and type 2 diabetes could be key triggers of DISH, leading to bone formation by targeting cells in the soft tissue ligaments and tendons, causing their proliferation and ossification. However, few studies on the aetiology of DISH have been undertaken and the hypothesis remains unproven. Nonetheless, due to the consistent association between DISH, obesity and hyperinsulinaemia, DISH is now seen by some researchers as associated with metabolic syndrome, perhaps co-occurring with obesity because of a shared mechanism of inflammation. It is predicted to rise in future Western European populations.

HFI

Hyperostosis Frontalis Interna (HFI) is also a condition whose aetiology has remained elusive and likewise little medical research has been carried out into it due to its lack of clinical significance. HFI consists of an overgrowth of bone on the endocranial (inner) surface of the frontal bone of the cranium and presents as undulating or lobulated bony protuberances (Fig. 131). These bony outgrowths are thought to develop in response to increased vascularisation or revascularisation (angiogenesis or the formation of new blood vessels) of the soft tissue layer attaching the frontal bone (dura).

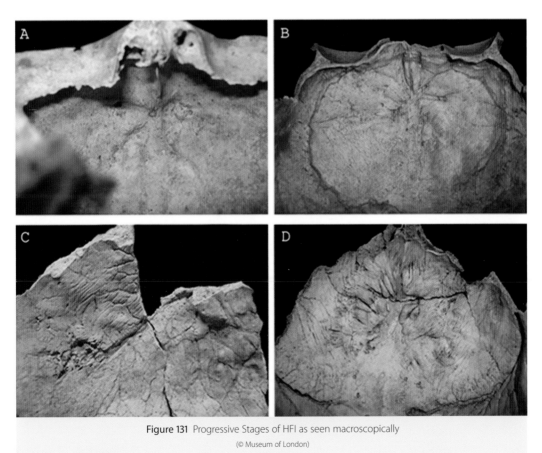

Figure 131 Progressive Stages of HFI as seen macroscopically
(© Museum of London)

Current research into HFI carried out at the Museum of London suggests that it is likely to be linked to metabolic syndrome, as is thought to be the case with DISH. Indeed, previous research has found that there is a tendency for HFI and DISH to co-occur and that hyperinsulinaemia can occur with HFI. One major difference between DISH and HFI is that HFI is predominantly found in post-menopausal women and its aetiology has therefore been linked to sex hormones. HFI is a progressive condition but its prevalence rates in the 50+ years age groups reaches a plateau, which follows a similar pattern to the production of testosterone by the ovaries in post-menopausal females (Fig. 132). Severe HFI in post-menopausal women is frequently accompanied by obesity and hyperandrogenism, an excessive level of androgens (male hormones) in the female body. As we have seen, excess weight leads to inflammation causing dysregulation of insulin from excessive levels of free fatty acids in addition to dysregulation of the sex hormones from the associated reduction of SHBG production by the liver. In women, this excess insulin also leads to slightly but significantly elevated ovarian testosterone production. The excess testosterone, unlike the case with obese men, stimulates a cycle of increased obesity (in particular visceral adipose tissue), increased free androgens, and decreased SHBG levels, all of which contribute towards hyperandrongenism and metabolic syndrome.

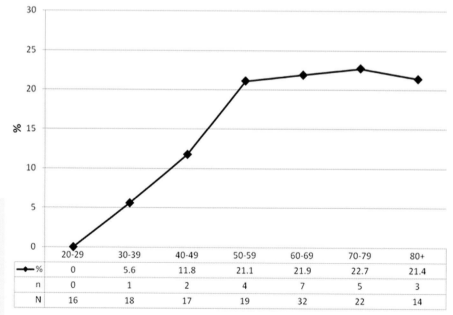

Figure 132
HFI prevalence rates according to age group in females (Christchurch Spitalfields and St Bride's Crypt assemblages combined)
(Western and Bekvalac 2017)

	20-29	30-39	40-49	50-59	60-69	70-79	80+
%	0	5.6	11.8	21.1	21.9	22.7	21.4
n	0	1	2	4	7	5	3
N	16	18	17	19	32	22	14

Decennial Age Categories

The mechanism behind angiogenesis in HFI and its skeletal manifestation in the frontal bone may be driven by metabolic syndrome acting in tandem with increased androgens in females. Androgen receptor (AR) is activated by binding to free androgens and can be stimulated by the growth factors IGF-1 and insulin associated with hyperinsulinaemia. AR is well established as a critical component of angiogenesis. For example, AR expression in certain diseases, such as prostate carcinoma, induces the production the fibroblast growth factors (FGFs), which are regulators of angiogenesis. It has been observed that the frontal bones have a higher sensitivity to FGFs than the other cranial bones but currently no studies have been undertaken to establish whether a similar mechanism of AR induced FGF production operates in HFI.

Another observation is that AR immunoreactivity is expressed by CD34 positive stem cells and fibroblasts in the vascular system. CD34 is an antigen that is present in

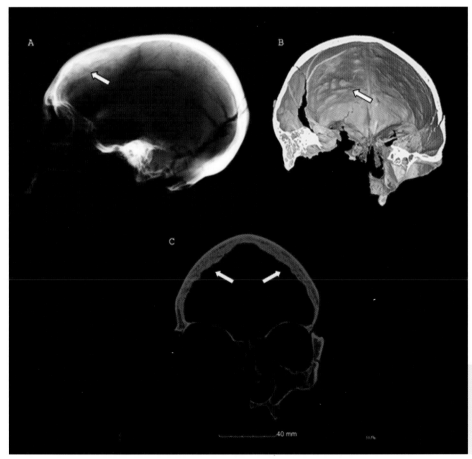

Figure 133 HFI identification using radiographic (A) and CT scanning (B and C) analysis
(© Museum of London)

vascular-associated cells undergoing differentiation and reproduction, and therefore can be used as a marker to evaluate angiogenesis. CD34 reactivity has been noted in dural fibroblasts in fibrous tumours but again, no clinical studies have to been undertaken to date to demonstrate whether cells present in HFI lesions are CD34 reactive. Since testosterone is the source of oestrogen in post-menopausal females, it is also possible that oestrogen and vascular endothelial growth factor (VEGF) also play a role in angiogenesis in HFI.

Rates of HFI in post-menopausal women in modern populations have been reported as being between 40 and 60%, and in 5–12% of the general population overall. To date, there have been few cases of consistent recording of HFI in archaeological skeletons due to its location within the cranium; if a cranium is complete, it is not possible to observe the inner surface of the frontal bone without endoscopic or radiographic examination. Fortunately, HFI can be seen quite clearly on radiographs, since it causes a distinct increased density to the frontal bone (Fig. 133).

Changes in metabolic syndrome over time

We examined a total of 1872 crania using radiography in order to detect the presence of HFI in our pre-Industrial and industrial period populations from London and areas outside the City (Table 15). The majority of cases (58.2%) were found in old aged females with a further 16.4% of cases affecting middle aged females. Only 9.1% and 7.2% of cases were found in old aged and middle aged males respectively.

Among old aged females, the highest rate of HFI was present in the Industrial period group from London (13.3%). This was followed by a rate of 9.7% in the Industrial period group from outside of London. The lowest rates of HFI were in the pre-Industrial old age females, where no cases were found in London and only 4.5% from outside of London were affected. Overall, the rates of HFI in the old aged females from London were not significantly higher than their contemporaries from outside London during either the Industrial or pre-Industrial periods, even when middle aged females were included in the sample. However, there was a significant increase in HFI over time from the pre-industrial to the Industrial period, for the old age female group as well as middle and old aged female groups combined. The combined data indicate that rates of HFI were almost four and a half times higher in the Industrial period, rising from 2.2% to 9.7%.

Looking at the Industrial period data from London in more detail, there is a significantly higher rate of HFI in high status old aged females (17.9%) than in lower status old aged females (8.1%). The social status of old aged females within

Table 15 HFI prevalence rates according to age and group in female (F) and male (M) adults according to age (YA = young adult, MA = middle adult and OA = old adult)

	FYA	FMA	FOA	MYA	MMA	MOA	Total
HFI cases	2	2	28	0	3	5	40
Industrial London	159	106	211	91	105	176	848
%	1.3	1.9	13.3	0	2.9	2.8	4.7
HFI cases	1	5	3	0	1	0	10
Industrial non-metropolitan	68	42	31	63	74	72	350
%	1.5	11.9	9.7	0	1.4	0	2.9
HFI cases	1	1	0	0	0	0	2
Pre-Industrial London	104	45	23	104	84	38	398
%	1.0	2.2	0	0	0	0	0.5
HFI cases	1	1	1	0	0	0	3
Pre-Industrial non-metropolitan	66	44	22	57	46	41	276
%	1.5	2.3	4.5	0	0	0	1.1
HFI cases	5	9	32	0	4	5	55
Total	397	237	287	315	309	327	1872
%	1.3	3.8	11.1	0	1.3	1.5	2.9

the London group therefore had a considerable effect on prevalence of HFI in the Industrial period. High status old aged female Londoners had the highest prevalence rates of HFI than any of the other groups.

In order to examine rates of DISH in the past, we collected data from a total of 3045 archaeological skeletons in which the mid-lower thoracic spine was present (Table 16). Overall, DISH mirrored the trends seen with HFI, increasing over time and with age, although primarily affecting old age males rather than females as expected. Of the total number of observed cases of DISH, 56.1% occurred in old adult males with a further 27.3% occurring in middle aged males. Only 7.9% and 3.6% of cases occurred in old aged and middle aged females respectively.

Comparable rates of the DISH were seen in the Industrial period old aged males from London (15.2%) and outside of London (16.1%), which were higher than pre-Industrial levels in both populations (11.5% and 9.6%) respectively. Combining the data for middle aged and old aged males, there was a significant increase in the rates of DISH over time from the pre-industrial (7.9%) to the industrial period (12.0%) but this rise did not occur equally in the City and locations beyond. In fact, prevalence rates of DISH in pre-Industrial and Industrial London amongst middle and old aged males were almost the same (10.0% compared to 10.7%), showing almost no change over time. Outside of London, however, rates of DISH in these age groups more than doubled from 6.3% to 14.3% over the same period (Fig. 134).

Table 16 DISH Prevalence Rates according to age and group

	FYA	FMA	FOA	MYA	MMA	MOA	Total
DISH cases	0	0	6	0	6	41	53
Industrial London	197	129	249	131	170	269	1145
%	0	0	2.4	0	3.5	15.2	4.6
DISH cases	1	4	4	2	16	18	45
Industrial non-metropolitan	104	82	66	100	126	112	590
%	1.0	4.9	6.1	2.0	12.7	16.1	7.6
DISH cases	0	0	0	1	12	7	20
Pre-Industrial London	141	88	39	161	129	61	619
%	0	0	0	0.6	9.3	11.5	3.2
DISH cases	1	1	1	3	4	12	22
Pre-Industrial non-metropolitan	132	92	88	125	129	125	691
%	0.8	1.1	1.1	2.4	3.1	9.6	3.2
DISH cases	2	5	11	5	38	78	139
Total	574	391	442	517	554	567	3045
%	0.3	1.3	2.5	1.0	6.9	13.8	4.6

Comparing the high status to low status middle and old aged males, there was a significantly higher rate of DISH amongst the high status males (19.3%) compared to those from low status areas (5.5%) (Fig. 134). There was even more of a contrast between old aged males alone, with rates of DISH being 23.4% compared to 8.3%. As with HFI, social status played a key role in DISH prevalence, with Industrial Period high status middle and old aged male Londoners having the highest rate of DISH compared to the other groups.

Overall, the age profile of DISH and HFI in past populations corresponds well to that of metabolic syndrome observed in modern populations, though the total prevalence rates are below the reported 30% of old age adults affected in Europe today. Further research is needed to identify precisely how many people in modern populations with metabolic syndrome have DISH or HFI and vice versa. Combining the evidence from DISH and HFI, an average of 14.6% of old age adults were affected by either condition during the Industrial period, whereas the rate was just 8.6% in the pre-Industrial population. The skeletal evidence suggests that rates of DISH and HFI, and the likely associated metabolic syndrome including obesity and hyperinsulinaemia, have increased over time but that these increases have affected males and females differently according to their social status and where they lived. DISH in male Londoners appears consistently over time whereas for males outside

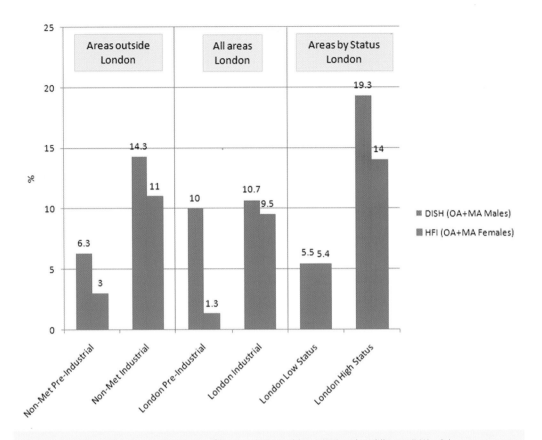

Figure 134 Comparative rates of DISH and HFI in old age (OA) and middle age (MA) adults

of London, the rates have increased substantially from the pre-Industrial to the Industrial periods. For females, rates of HFI have increased significantly over time irrespective of location. By the Industrial periods, both males and females of high status have the highest rates of metabolic DISH or HFI.

In other words, London was a tale of two cities. It has consistently had its fair share of high status fat cat males throughout but it appears that only by the Industrial period did wealthy women catch up with their counterparts in the excesses of food, drink and leisurely lifestyles. In comparison, both men and women from outside of the City were equally tardy in earning their place at the table. Low status males and females in the City seldom got the opportunity to take a seat. Rates of these potential metabolic syndrome skeletal manifestations were consistently higher than in males than in females, though low status males and females were almost equally affected.

Patty cake, patty cake, baker man: hospitality in the city

London has a long history featuring hospitality and the food trade (Fig. 135). William Fitz Stephen in around 1173 wrote of the City

'If any of the citizens should unexpectedly receive visitors weary from their journey, who would fain not wait until fresh food is brought and cooked, or until servants have brought bread...they hasten to the river bank and there find all they need. However great the multitude of soldiers and travellers entering the city, or preparing to go out of it, at any hour of the day or night – that these may not fast too long, and those may not go out supperless – they turn aside thither, if they please, where every man can refresh himself in his own way.'

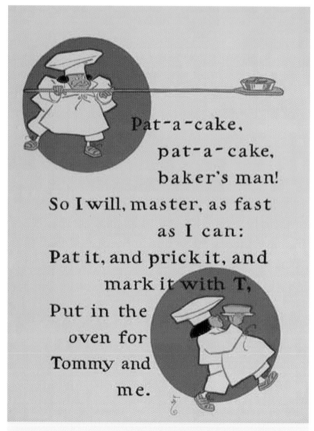

Figure 135 Original copyright 1902 by William Wallace Denslow in *Mother Goose*. The earliest written reference of the rhyme dates to 1698

(Project Gutenberg EBook, http://www.gutenberg.org/etex, PD Gutenberg)

This is the first historical record of London's fast food joints, or cookshops, located along the Thames riverbank between Queenhithe and Dowgate, serving their cosmopolitan clientele with hot dishes of meat, fish and poultry to suit all budgets. In fact, the history of cooks in London goes back a little further. The *Worshipful Company of Cooks* in London's origins date to 1170 following the amalgamation of two pre-existing guilds: the *Cooks of Eastcheap* and the *Cooks of Bread Street*. Over the course of the next couple of centuries, the fast food industry boomed as the City grew and, by the late 13th and early 14th centuries, there were specialist bakers, flan makers, pastelers (pastry cooks), cheesemongers, saucers, waferers and mustard sellers all catering to this developing market. The streets of Westminster and London, including Cheapside, Candlewick Street, Friday Street, 'Pottage Island' at St Martin-in-the-Fields, 'Pie Corner' at Smithfield and Eastcheap, were bustling with every kind of food seller and hawkers, crying out and advertising their wares with, 'Hot pies, hot! Good piglets and geese, go dine, go!'

This was in contrast to small towns and villages, though the evolution of cookshops stems from the same origin. Traditionally, in medieval villages, corn was taken to the village mill for grinding into flour or meal. Many houses were not furnished with their own kitchens or ovens to bake food. Even in towns like Colchester, for example, only 3% of taxpaying households were noted as having a kitchen. Additionally, there were issues in keeping meat fresh. Instead, it was commonplace for food and bread to be cooked by the village baker, to whom people took their own dough, meat and raw foodstuffs. This practice continued both in villages and urban centres into at least the 19th century and was a shared practice between both people of wealth and those of limited means. However, the expansion of urban centres of trade demanding an increase in labour led to a high percentage of migrants and labourers in the cities. This was especially the case in London, where often single males living in shared accommodation and had no access to cooking facilities. This led to an ever-growing demand for ready-made food on the go, especially hot food. Cookshops rapidly became a vital source of cheap hot food for the poor and vulnerable living in meagre housing, with or without providing the raw ingredients. The demand for cooks in the City rose accordingly. In Southwark alone where 41% of the population consisted of single men and women, there were 16 bakers, cooks and pie bakers between 1377 and 1381. In comparison, the same records indicate that the whole of Worcester only had three bakers and no cooks at all, likely due to the much lower presence of only 13% of single men or women.

Slap-bang shops

The provision of meat, whether roasted, fried or boiled, was quintessentially the role of cookshops and chop-shops, or 'slap-bang shops' as they were known (Fig. 136). Early cookshops by the river in London in Cooks Row are described by Michael Symons as being furnished with, 'generally four spits, one over the another, carry around each five or six pieces of butcher's meat, beef, mutton, veal, pork and lamb; you have what quantity you please cut off fat, lean, much or little done. With this, a little salt and mustard upon the side of a plate, a bottle of beer and a roll'. London eateries in 1786 were described as a place 'you walk in as you would into a public space – freely and without fuss' in contrast to dining out in Paris where the formalities of dining in public were much stricter. Standards at cookshops varied however, particularly when serving the cheapest pies for the lower working classes, often labourers, mechanics, hackney coachmen, sedan

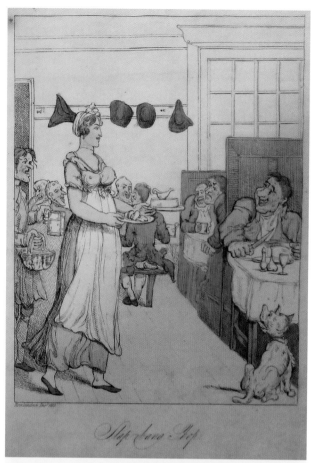

Figure 136 *The interior of an Eating-house. All the customers look round to smile expectantly at a tall and comely young woman who enters alluringly from the left, carrying dishes. She is followed by a small man with two tankards and a basket. Tables on the right are divided by high settles. On the left men sit on benches at a long table. In the foreground sits a dog looking round hungrily.* 1815

(public domain)

chairmen and footmen. Many had a bad reputation for the providing reheated meats and serving 'measly pork, rusty bacon, stinking lamb, rotten mutton, coddled cow, yellow greens and sooty pottage' from suffocating steam-ridden basement shops. In 1699, Ned Ward, satirist and author of *The London Spy*, wrote that he was put off buying from a cookshop when he noticed the cook wiping his ears, forehead and armpits with the same damp cloth he applied to his pork!

Nonetheless, the importance of the cookshop in its provision of meat to the poor was still recognised in 1832 by the newly founded constabulary, who although highly desiring the closure of street markets and public houses to prevent drunk and disorderliness on Sundays, were supportive of the continued opening of cookshops to provide the poor with food. In Spitalfields, although the market was regularly open until midnight for working classes to purchase meat for Sunday's meal, it was understood that many might not have the facilities to keep it fresh or to cook it without access to a cookshop. The same was true of bread. By the Industrial period, cookshops in the working class areas had become a facility largely for serving the urban poor, whereby speed and convenience of the provision of cheap food was key for sustaining the labour force. In Spitalfields alone, witnesses at this time estimated that between 600 and 900 people were fed daily by the cookshops there. It was also noted that the free time afforded to the working classes on Sunday afternoon by buying ready-made food meant that they then could spend time walking about the fields around Bethnal Green and Hackney to get some fresh air and respite from the City.

Dining out in style

Certainly those who indulge in excess are much worse off in point of bodily health than others who are regular and steady.

Mr George Wilson, Resident of Tothill Street, Westminster, 1832.

Large feasts celebrating saints' days had been a long practised tradition but the very finest of banquets offering vast quantities of exquisite and luxury foods were reserved purely for the highest nobility, an excess of foodstuffs being a potent symbol of wealth and power. As the rigid social classes based solely on inheritance began to break down, self-made wealthy businessmen began to emulate these traditions (Fig. 137). A core theme of the Industrial period is its emphasis on material wealth and consumerism,

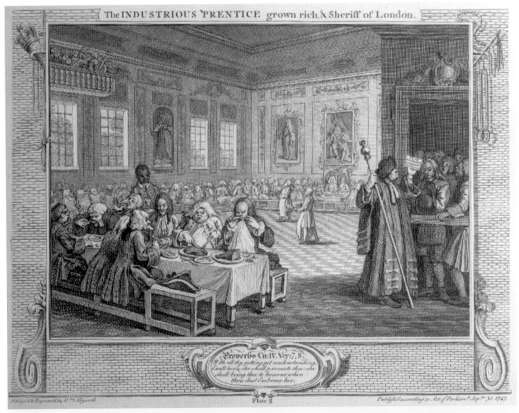

Figure 137 Engraving by Thomas Cook after William Hogarth, 1796, *Illustration of a banquet at the Fishmongers' Hall, Francis Goodchild, now Sheriff of London, and his wife, framed by a sword and mace, preside over a grand banquet. Sitting at a table in the foreground various dignitaries gorge themselves contrasting with the poor petitioners waiting at the door* (Wellcome Collection, cc-by/4.0)

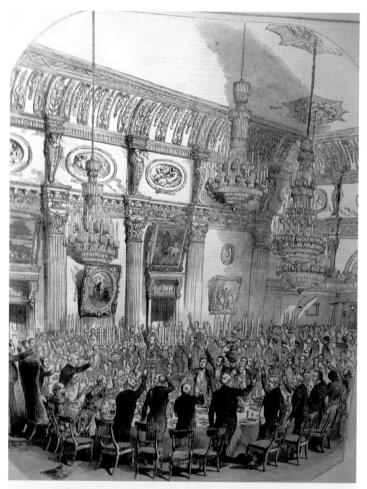
Figure 138 Illustration of the *London Tavern*, 19th century
(Ivan Day, http://foodhistorjottings.blogspot.com/2012/11/tavern-feasting-in-bristol-christmas.html © Ivan Day)

driving competitive trading: London by the 18th century was the busiest port in the world. Industrial expansion created new markets for exotic foods and goods, changing consumption and trading patterns. Both the consumption and bestowing of food with extravagant largesse were vehicles for acquiring social esteem and wealth. For the rising middle class men of position and influence, dining out as part of a social opportunity to advance business relationships became a popular activity during the 17th and 18th centuries. Coffee houses, originally established in Oxford and then appearing first in London in 1652 in St Michael's Alley, Cornhill, have been described as 'centres of political intrigue and commercial intelligence, as well as, primarily, dining rooms' by Michael Symons. Catering diversified into well-furnished eating-houses to meet this demand, where meals were served to the table accompanied by liquid refreshment such as ale or wine: the business lunch for commercial men, politicians and City clerks was born.

Taverns still offered to cook meals from raw ingredients bought buy their wealthy patrons (Fig. 138). Samuel Pepys, for example, bought a lobster from the local market in Fish Street and his friends bought a sturgeon, which they then took to the *Sun Tavern* to be cooked and served to them. In 1842, Charles Knight describes the quantity of meat prepared by the 200 or so eating houses in London as 'quite enormous', presenting a 'never-ceasing picture of eating and drinking'. In particular, he notes the haste with which the diners in the City frequent their eating-houses compared to those in Covent Garden and the Haymarket, most commonly frequented by actors, artisans, writers and tourists. Meals very often consisted of a platter of a variety of foods including meat, vegetables and cheese, sometimes served over three courses and priced accordingly. The excesses of London dining had been remarked upon earlier by George Cheyne (1672–1743). He blamed his move to the City at the beginning of the 18th century for his newly acquired obesity (Fig. 139). Socialising with the 'younger Gentry and Free-Livers', Cheyne describes himself as growing 'daily in bulk ... [and] excessively fat, short-breathed, Lethargic and Listless'. He moved to the country, changing his dietary regimen to a much restricted vegetarian diet, and lost his excess pounds.

The male and somewhat vulgar environment of these eating-houses provided no opportunity for women of social standing to dine out, especially if unaccompanied. Indeed, eating out up to this point was seen as such a red-blooded affair that there was great concern that any innovative luxury accompanying dining out might be emasculating, dulling the appetites and encouraging dandyism. Even among the working classes, though more out of necessity than desire, the paltry quantity of meat that could be afforded was purchased and cooked by the wife but consumed by the working husband. However, the increasing popularity of dining out among the middle classes, as became convenient to day trippers and shoppers in town, as well as the introduction of drinking tea with meals rather than beer, led to a more refined dining experience. French-style restaurants and later elegant soup-rooms with diners seated at separate tables started to be fashionable and by 1842 offered rooms where ladies could dine freely 'without any restraint from the observation of male visitors'. This new fashion and acceptance of ladies eating in public was closely tied to a newly imported food that was taken up with great zeal: sugar.

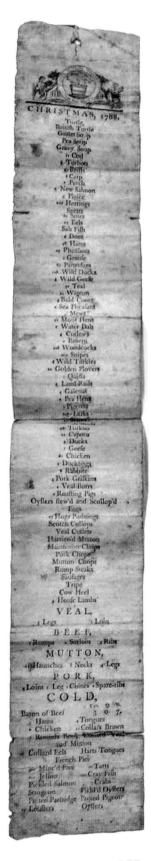

Figure 139 Bill of Fare (Menu) for Christmas 1788 from the *Bush Inn and Tavern*, Cornhill, Bristol

(Ivan Day http://foodhistorjottings.blogspot.com/2012/11/tavern-feasting-in-bristol-christmas.html © Ivan Day)

A taste for sweet success

Though the first historical reference to the presence of sugar in England dates to the 12th century, like all exotic foodstuffs, it had a very restricted use by a limited number of people. Principally it was used as a medicine, spice condiment or a decorative material, whereas honey was used traditionally as a sweetener. Sugar was an expensive item for the wealthy. Having been displaced by the Earl of Worcester at a banquet in 1464, the mayor of London was sent a' doggy-bag' to make amends for this social *faux pas*. It contained meat, bread, wine and 'many divers confections in sugar' to ensure that the offering conveyed sufficient splendour. New colonial mercantile endeavours based on slave exploitation and plantation development in the Caribbean ensured, however, that between 1630 and 1680, the retail price of sugar was halved (Fig. 140). The new agro-industry, ushering in the later Industrial Revolution within the country, created consumer demand for a previously unobtainable foodstuff by making large quantities available at decreased cost to the customer.

After 1660, sugar imports were enumerated for the purposes of tax. Though initially all annual imports of sugar from the Caribbean were subsequently exported

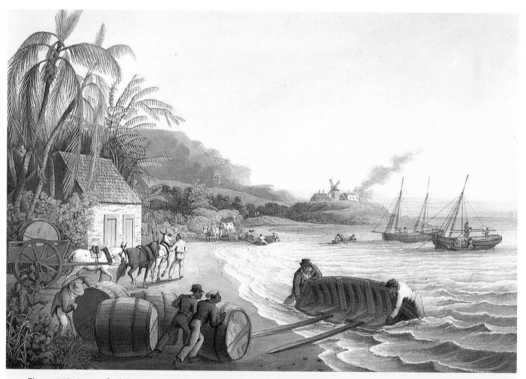

Figure 140 A prettified illustration of slaves loading barrels of sugar (sugar hogsheads) onto a boat, Antigua, 1823
(British Library Online/Flickr Commons)

out of Britain, the taste for sugar in the UK caught on quickly (Fig. 141). By 1753, only around 5% of imported sugar was being exported, 95% being consumed within the British Isles. Consumption of sugar over this period is estimated to have risen 20 fold, increasing more rapidly per capita than bread, meat or dairy items. By 1800, consumption is estimated to have risen by 2500% over 150 years and was set to rise even further. We see evidence of this reflected in

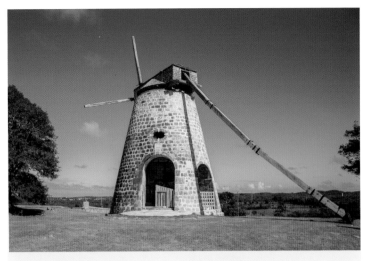

Figure 141 Old sugar mill in Antigua and Barbuda at Betty's Hope Sugar Plantation (Shutterstock.com)

archaeological skeletal remains. Prevalence rates of dental caries caused by sucrose almost doubled from 9.9% in pre-industrial London to 18.8% in the Industrial period.

In contrast to meat, sugar was very much associated with female consumption, ladies being cited as the 'patronesses of the fair sugar' by Dr Frederick Slare in 1715, since 'they had more experience and liberal use of it'. Dr Slare firmly believed that the female palate was more refined than men's tastes for 'tobacco, beer, salt and pickles' and furthermore, was something of a panacea, the only ill effects being 'that it could make ladies too fat'. Females had significantly higher rates of dental caries than males in Industrial period London, though this division between the sexes was not present in the pre- Industrial period. In spite of the discovery of diabetes mellitus by his rival academic Dr Willis around 1674, who suspected that sugar contained an acid corrosive salt that could have caused the disease, its popularity did not decline. Instead, the intertwined usage of sugar as a sweetener in tea, for those of more refined tastes, made it even more popular. In contrast to the somewhat raucous eating-houses, the advent of confectioners and tea gardens of the late 18th century offered a sophisticated atmosphere, where unaccompanied ladies of status could spend some of their newly acquired leisure time to stop and purchase delicacies such as pastries, sugar plums, comfits, jellies, creams and bonbons (Fig. 142). Not only that, a much wider variety of cooked foods, especially puddings, now contained sugar as an essential ingredient and became integral parts of the dining experience.

As the demand for sugar continued to grow, though still largely restricted to

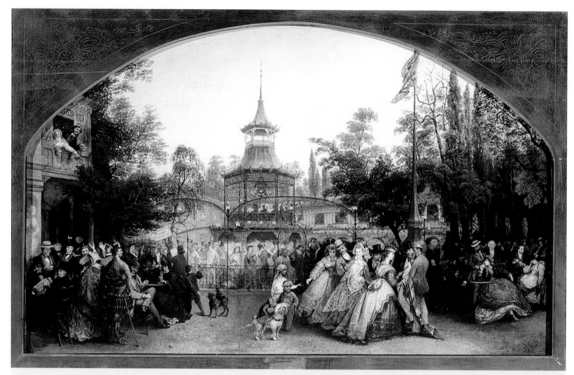

Figure 142 *The Dancing Platform at Cremorne Gardens, Chelsea, London,* by Phoebus Levin, 1864
(© Museum of London)

those of means as a luxury item, around 1850 free trade vanquished the monopoly held under the *Navigation Acts* over the import of sugar from the Caribbean. Free trade was aimed at reducing taxation on foreign sugar in order to raise monies from increased sales of what was by now an important economic commodity. At the same time, cheaper beet sugar became available for the first time due to the development of factory scale extraction on the Continent. Sugar prices dropped as dramatically as its consumption rose, as was true of tea. As a sweetener and preservative, it became a cheap source of calories for the working classes whose calorific intake was otherwise somewhat stunted. As sugar swamped the market, its importance as a social symbol of elegance and high status vanished (Fig. 143). Instead it became a foodstuff of vulgarity to be shunned for the associated tainted morality attributed to its new lowly consumers; 'by the notorious fact of the obesity of those who grow old in their vile trade and who gradually become positive monsters of adipose tissue', as Lombroso remarked of prostitutes in 1898.

Sugar had become an even greater component of diet from around 1875 by its use in cheap mass-produced jam and treacle. The diet of Lancashire operatives in 1864, typical of our Swinton population for example, was recorded by Edward Smith as consisting mainly of bread, oatmeal, bacon, a very small amount of butter, treacle, tea and coffee. Though a very healthy diet of cheap vegetables and fruits such as watercress, onions, carrots, turnips, cabbage, apples, gooseberries, plums, greengages and cherries were frequently purchased and consumed, the highly calorific bread and jam became a mainstay meal, particularly when women started working in factories and had much less time at home for food preparation.

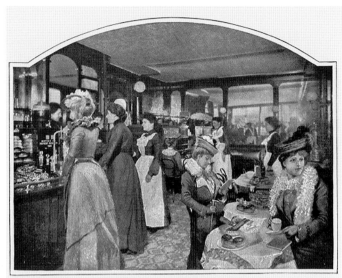

A WELL-KNOWN CONFECTIONER'S SHOP (PICCADILLY).

Figure 143 From *Living London* by George R Sims, 1902
(https://archive.org/details/livinglondonitsw02sims)

Sugar consumption soared: from the reasonably insignificant amount of 4 lb (1.8 kg) of sugar per annum per person in 1700, consumption by 1900 was 60 lb (27.2 kg).

Examination of the osteoarchaeological data offers an interesting perspective here, however. The evidence indicates that there was a significantly higher prevalence rate of caries among females of low social status than those of high status, reflecting their increased consumption of sugar. However, we have also seen that HFI, associated with obesity and hyperinsulinaemia, was conversely significantly higher in females of higher status, suggesting that despite the lower rate of sugar intake, more high status females were overweight. This is explained by the pure level of labour intensive work undertaken by low status individuals as part of the daily grind. Victorian working class males and females are estimated to have required 3000–4500 and 2750–3500 calories a day respectively, 50–100% more calories on average than today. In contrast, although their sugar consumption may have been lower, high status ladies would have done comparatively little exercise and would have had to moderate their calorific intake to control their weight. Evidently, for some, the sweet temptation was just too much and this is a trend that has continued over time alongside our increasingly sedentary lifestyles.

Palm oil and fatty acids

The use of food additives as a preserver in order to prolong shelf life and sell cheap mass-produced food has continued to be a successful strategy by manufacturers of convenience foods. Today, palm oil is a top product used by most of the fast food chains on the high street, either as a key ingredient or for frying foods. Though the history of importing palm oil into the British Isles dates back to at least the 16th and 17th centuries, initially being traded via caravans and ships of the Atlantic slave trade and subsequently imported from central Africa during the Industrial period (Fig. 144) for use in candle making and as a lubricant for machines, the demand for palm oil has grown exponentially in recent years due to its manifold uses.

Like sugar, rates of consumption of palm oil have soared. From 2009 to 2014 alone, British imports have risen from 155,000 metric tonnes to just over 396,109 metric tonnes, according to DEFRA. It has become popular with manufacturers because it is much cheaper than alternative oils, being much higher in yield and requiring less land for a higher output. Palm oil is naturally composed of fatty acids and has a very high concentration of saturated fat. In modern usage, palm oil is refined to create many foods and household products but as a result of this process, it contains a contaminant called glycidyl fatty acid esters (GE). Rice and palm oil form the highest levels of GE during not only the refinement process but also from use in frying, barbecuing and baking, where palm oil contains 4–12% of the precursor of GE. When consumed, GE is converted into free fatty acid in the gastrointestinal tract, causing

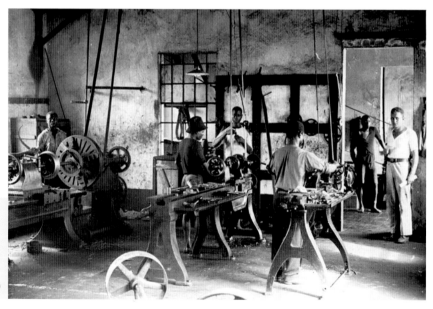

Figure 144 Palm oil works, *c.* 1900, Cameroon, Central Africa.

(Bundesarchiv, Bild 137-034031/cc-by-sa/3.0, https://de.wikipedia.org/wiki/Datei:Bundesarchiv_Bild_137-034031,_Kamerun,_Palm%C3%B6lwerk_Bota.jpg)

cancer in rodents; as such, GE is classified as a 'possible human carcinogen' by the International Agency for Research on Cancer (IARC).

Of equal concern is the identification of a specific protein known as CD36 located in the cell membranes of tumour cells in oral tumours, melanoma skin cancer, ovarian, bladder, lung and breast cancer. This protein takes up fatty acids and initiates metastasis. Palmitic acid, not only a major component of palm oil but also present in meat and dairy products, has been tested on CD36 and was found to double the rate of oral cancer metastasis in mice. Conversely, CD36 blocking antibodies significantly reduced 80–90% of the metastases. Fatty acids are also synthesised by fatty acid synthase (FASN). Cancer cells of the breast, prostate, colon, ovary, endometrium and thyroid express high levels of FASN and upregulated metabolism of fatty acids are linked to the proliferation of cancer cells. Initial research also suggests that fatty acids from palmitic acid may lead to DNA damage as well as to compromised DNA damage response during the transition to cancer cell formation. The balance of healthy fatty acids in the body is shifted towards an accumulation of palmitic acids by excessive intake of carbohydrates, a sedentary life style and overeating.

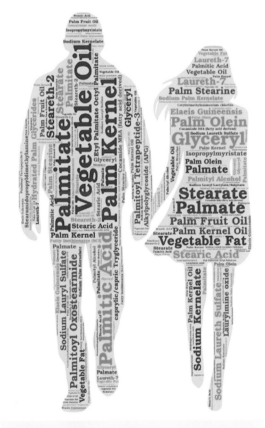

Despite the evidence for the potential harm that refined edible oils such as palm oil have on the body, the demand for palm oil continues to increase and currently approximately half of all packaged products sold in supermarkets contain palm oil. Common items of processed products containing palmitic acid include cosmetics, toothpaste, instant noodles, shampoo, ice cream, margarine, peanut butter, chocolate bars, soap and bread, though the list is by no means exhaustive. Given the direct link to cancer, a diet of processed and high fat foods is to be avoided. However, of concern is the lack of clear labelling: Green Palm who certificate sustainable sources of palm oil, has identified 36 different labels for palm oil and its derivatives (Fig. 145), making it difficult for consumers to identify exactly what they are eating.

Figure 145 Different labels for palm oil and its derivatives
(G. Western)

Consumption, obesity and health today

Looking back at the history of British dietary health, a remarkable picture of emerges of the interdependence between social aspirations, commerce and food consumption which invariably leaves its mark on the human body. As the leading capital at the centre of international sugar trade (Fig. 146), London's imports mirrored and directed the dynamics of social behaviour regarding dietary traditions and customs. Its cosmopolitan environment in conjunction with its strong drive towards consumerism necessitated a wide range of public hospitality venues, which developed from the more traditional role of providing sustenance for the local populace and diverged in nature according to the status of their clientele. As time went on, the over-riding demand for speed and convenience demanded by industrialism quickly became the norm in urban populace across the county. This requirement has reached almost fever pitch in the UK today, with networks of fast food outlets, restaurants, shops and supermarkets selling convenience foods within walking distance in every town and city.

Over recent years, the increased use of food additives such as sugar and palm oil has created a decrease in the market for fresh ingredients, regular components of diet bought on a daily basis until the advent of packaged convenience food, and an increase in obesity, diabetes and dental caries (Fig. 147). The consumption of sugar in Britain per person per year is now estimated at 150 lb (68 kg). Currently, around 3.4

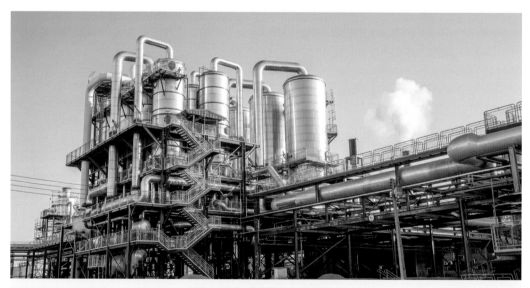

Figure 146 Sugar refining factory, US
(Shutterstock.com)

million people in the UK or 9% of the adults are estimated to have type 2 diabetes and approximately one-third of the adults have tooth decay. Hidden sugars, as they are now known, are causing such a cost to both human health and the budget of the NHS that the well-publicised sugar tax was introduced on drinks in 2018 to discourage manufacturers from including it in such high levels in their products. After only a few months, the financial penalties have had considerable impact on the production of high sugar soft drinks, incidentally also being expected to raise £275m per year in taxation revenue. The gravity of the impact of obesity for many still is not clear. One in 20 cases of cancer are contributed to by excess weight, which causes a total of 18,100 cancer cases a year in the UK; however, three-quarters of people asked in a recent survey did not think cancer could result from excess weight (Cancer Research UK).

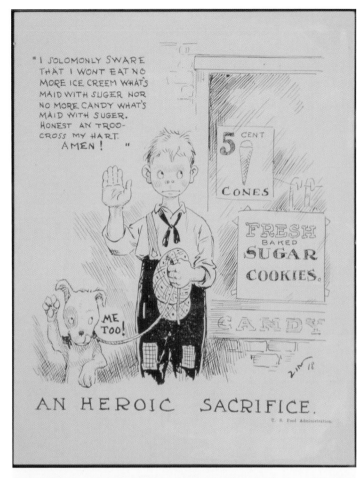

Figure 147 First World War Food Economy Poster, Education Division. *c.* 1917–1919
(National Archives, U.S. Food Administration. Educational Division, Advertising, World War I Posters, 512512, access unrestricted, https://catalog.archives.gov/id/512512)

Today, national economic development is still influential for obesity levels in concert with social status. In countries where comparative GDP is low, those of higher socio-economic status are more likely to be obese whereas in countries with high GDP, the reverse is true with lower rates of obesity in those of higher social status. A similar trend is found in the prevalence rates of dental caries today in England. The Adult Dental Health Survey in 2009 found that only 19% of people in managerial and professional occupations experienced tooth decay compared to 27% of people from routine and manual backgrounds. Today, many people of higher socio-economic

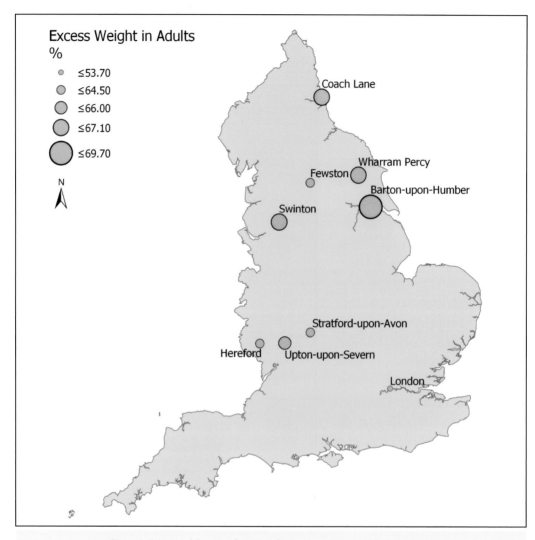

Figure 148 National Statistics for rates of excess weight according to location

status have cultural tastes and norms that dictate that an excess of food is to be eschewed, whereas in the past, largeness was a symbol of largesse among City's high status population.

The osteoarchaeological data appears to confirm recent assertions that as a nation, we have never been so fat. However, according to the data from Public Health England for 2015–6, rates of excess weight and diabetes in London are now much lower than in the areas outside of London. (Figs 148 and 149). The highest rate of excess weight according to BMI and diabetes outside of London was seen in the Barton-upon-Humber area at 7% and 69.7% respectively (NE Lincolnshire CCG)

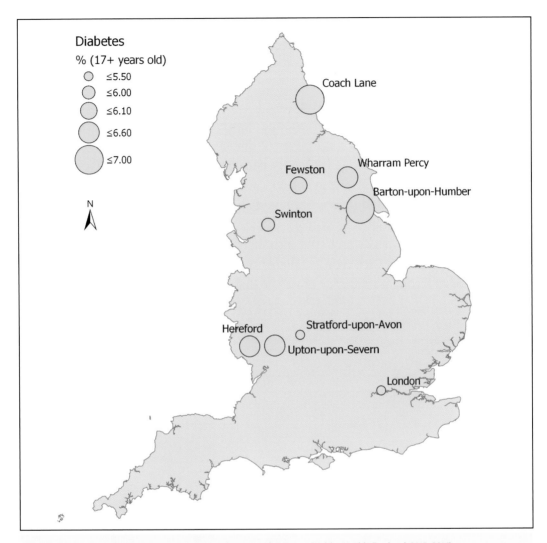

Figure 149 National statistics for rates of diabetes (Public Health England, 2015–2016)

whereas the lowest rates of 5.4% and 63.7% respectively was in Stratford-upon-Avon (South Warwickshire CCG). Correspondingly, Barton-upon- Humber also had the higher percentage of physically inactive adults (27.4% v 23.9%), lower percentage of adults meeting the five-a-day fresh fruit and vegetables in their diets (49.5% v 60.1%) and had the higher deprivation score (30.9 v 11.6) compared to Stratford-upon-Avon. In London, increasing deprivation scores were strongly correlated with increasing prevalence rates of diabetes (Figs 150 and 151), with the exception of Brentford in outer London, which had one of the highest rates of diabetes and excess weight despite having the lowest deprivation score in the London area. Excluding Brentford, the highest rates of diabetes and excess weight in Inner London were recorded by Tower Hamlets CCG (6.8% and 52.5% respectively) in 2014–2015 compared to the lower rates of 4.3% and 47.3% respectively in Chelsea (West London and Kensington CCG).

Overall, the risk factors associated with diabetes, such as physical inactivity, excess weight, smoking and not eating five fresh fruit and vegetable portions a day are significantly associated with economic deprivation and social status. In fact, according to Public Health England, type 2 diabetes is 40% more common among people today in the least deprived category nationwide. This is a reversal of the trend observed in our past populations in London, where skeletal changes associated with metabolic syndrome, including obesity and diabetes, were found most frequently in high status groups.

Interesting to note is the fact that although according to the National Diabetes Audit data, 90% of adults with type 2 diabetes are overweight, excess weight measured by BMI is not as strong a predictor of risk of diabetes as raised waist circumference.

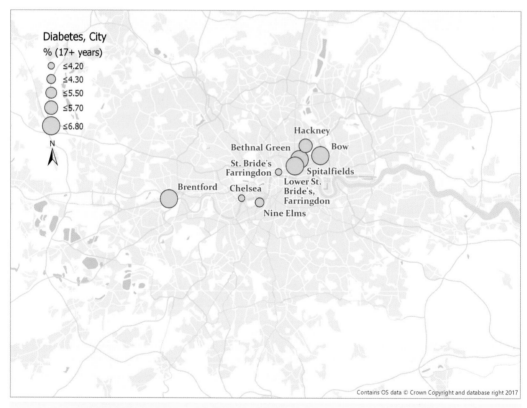

Figure 150 London statistics for rates of diabetes (Public Health England, 2015–2016)

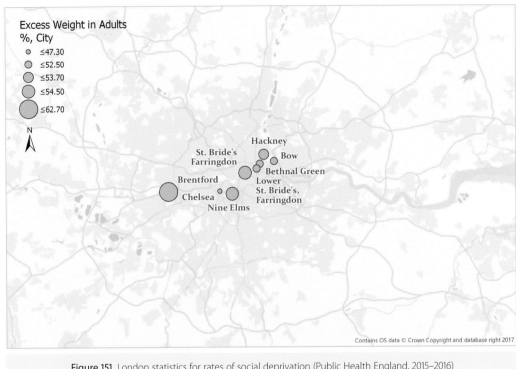

Figure 151 London statistics for rates of social deprivation (Public Health England, 2015–2016)

Across our groups, diabetes prevalence has only a moderately significant relationship with rates of premature death, excess weight and the relative number of inactive adults. This indicates that today, the relationship between these contributory factors is not always straightforward and suggests that the picture of obesity and its health implications is complex, with local cultural variations in diet, lifestyle, smoking, and social status at times having a conflicting influence on diabetes development. In addition, it is also estimated that 25% of people with type 2 diabetes are undiagnosed and so reported figures of diabetes are underestimates. What is clear is that there is a relationship between increasing age and higher diabetes rates. The National Institute for Health Care and Excellence (NICE) recognises that being older than 40 years is a significant risk factor for diabetes. The rate of diabetes in those aged over 75 years old was reported as 16.5% by Public Health England in 2014, compared to only 2% of individuals aged 16–24 years old and 5.1% of those aged 35–54 years old. This has serious future implications for our ageing population.

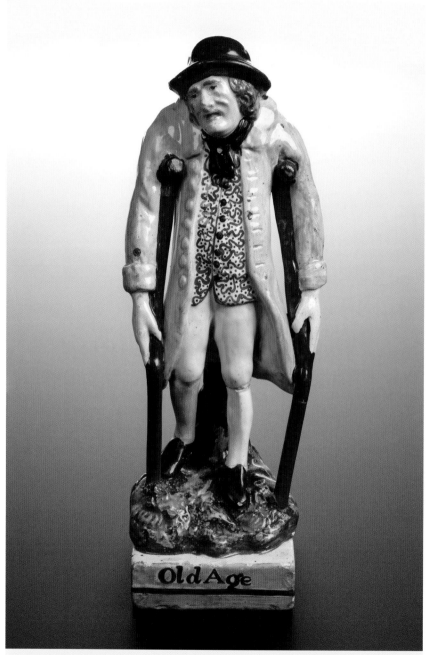

Figure 152 'Old Age' statue, Staffordshire, England, 1801–1830

(Science Museum, cc-by/4.0)

5

Getting old: us in winter clothes

Ageing is a complex passage, with many interlocking causes, from healthy youth to decline and death

The United Nations Population Fund (UNPF) has identified that ageing is a 'global phenomenon' and will be one of the most significant trends for the 21st century. Currently over 11% of the world's population are 60 years and older, predicted to rise to 22% by 2050 (UNFPA, 2002 and 2012). Senescence, the fact of becoming older, is a complex process. The causes of ageing are still not fully understood and remain an ever more pertinent focus for scientific investigations, such as The Baltimore Longitudinal Study of Aging, which began in 1958. At its core, it has the question 'What is normal ageing?' The scientific investigation of ageing and its associated risk factors for health, otherwise known as gerontology, is still seeking the answer to this question by examining the physical, cognitive and disease aspects of getting older.

The Office for National Statistics recorded that from 2014 to 2016, life expectancy at birth in the UK was 79.2 years for males and 82.9 years for females. It estimates from current trends that by 2066, people aged 85 years and over will make up 7% of the total UK population. The two-fold trend for both population ageing and population growth has steadily continued in the UK's recent history for both males and females, with the only dips in the last 100 years occurring at the times of the First and Second World Wars, followed by more rapid increases of growth from the 1950s onwards (Fig. 153).

Recent data from the Trust for London, however, showed that London's age structure is different to the rest of England, having a higher proportion of 25–34 year olds and a lower proportion of those aged 50+ and above. According to the 2011

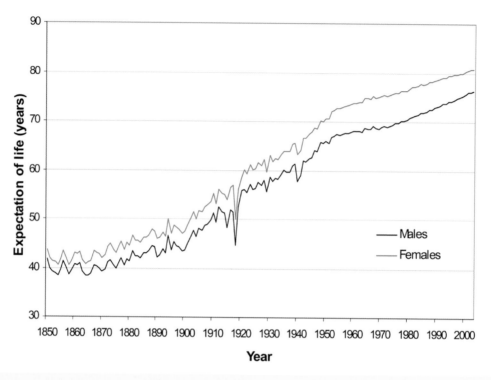

Figure 153 Expectation of life at birth, England and Wales, (1850–2003) taken from *Mortality Improvements and Evolution of Life Expectancies*

(A. Gallop)

census data, only 10% of households in Inner London and 16% in Outer London are pensioner households, compared to the 22% found in other areas of England. With this greater dominance of a younger population and often stark social variation between rich and poor, Harry Leslie Smith in an article in *The Guardian* highlighted the feeling of a loss of compassion for the old and an economic imbalance amongst London's senior citizens, with increasing loneliness and marginalisation of the elderly. To him, 'London without old people isn't a city, it's just a factory floor, with no history, no past or future, just an endless present tense in pursuit of money'.

Although life expectancy has increased over our recent past, it is unclear as to whether this is actually part of a continuing trend occurring over a long period of time and whether this differed according to location. So what has triggered our increasing old age and when did this start? What was old age in the past like and what were the implications then? Was growing old in London different to other areas of the UK in the past?

What is old age?

The construct of ageing has distinct meanings for different cultures and societies and as such, it is difficult to precisely define the meaning of old age. Age can be identified by:

- Your chronological age, as in how old you are in years
- Your biological age, in terms of your body and how it functions
- Your psychological age, relating to how old a person feels, acts and behaves
- Your social age, relating to the changing roles and relationships as a person ages

In terms of looking at age based upon a chronological conception, the United Nations identifies that 65 years is generally the agreed threshold that signifies old age. In many Western countries, about this age is also seen as the classification for retirement and being regarded as a senior citizen. In modern law, the term 'senior citizen' means that pensions and social benefits can be made available by the State for supporting the individual. In the UK, the first non-contributory pension paid for the elderly (individuals 70 years or older) came about from the *Pensions Act* in 1908, paying an amount of 5 shillings a week, in present day money worth about £25. There were various caveats for those who could receive the pension, notably that the man or woman had to be 70 or over, have been a British subject for at least 20 years, lived in the UK and their yearly means not to have exceeded £31. 10s. With none of the study sites excavated having a date parameter beyond the 1870s, the men and women included in this project would have had to find the means to support themselves in old age. For those coming from a wealthier background, there would be independent funds. Such individuals may have retired comfortably but many elderly individuals would have had to continue to work. Between 1851 and 1911, 86–93% of men aged 60 years old and over were still working and many of these were general or agricultural labourers. To die in harness was a familiar way of life.

For those living in poverty, this could well have meant needing support from the parish funds or perhaps being lucky enough to find a place at an almshouse. The Statute of Charitable Uses in 1601 was the first to make provision for 'the relief of the aged' and thereby explicitly marks the beginning of the use of almshouses for accommodating the elderly. The first post-Reformation private charity to support this movement was the Queen Elizabeth's College in Greenwich, London, where almshouses (Fig. 154) have been present since 1576 and to this day still provides housing for those over 65 years old in financial hardship. Most almshouses in the 19th century stipulated 50, 55 or 60 years as the threshold for entry as an old age person. However, almshouses very

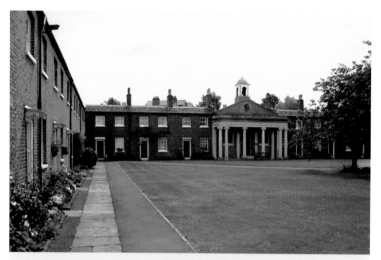

Figure 154 Almshouses at Queen Elizabeth's College in Greenwich, London
(© Hanover Anchor Housing Association, https://www.hanover.org.uk/ /queen-elizabeth-college-greenwich/)

often did not allow access to those in receipt of parish funds and following the *Poor Law Amendment Act* of 1834, many destitute would find themselves being faced with no option but to enter a workhouse.

Although perhaps more challenging to identify in the past, there was, as is a feature of society today, neglect of the elderly. Karen Chase notes in her book 'Victorians and Old Age' that in attempts to banish the elderly poor to institutions, terms such as 'old age', 'lunacy' and 'imbecility' were obscured and interchangeable. Most adults living in workhouses were old age. However, the vulnerability of old age people to workhouse submission differed according to sex and residential area. In locations outside of London, such as at Upton-on-Severn, Wharfedale (Fewston) and Hereford (Figs 155–157), old aged males were more vulnerable and were present in workhouses in relatively higher numbers

Figure 155 Age profile demographics comparing workhouse and general population from 1881 census data for Upton-upon-Severn (based on data from www.workhouses.org.uk) (YA = young adult, MA = middle adult and OA = old adult)

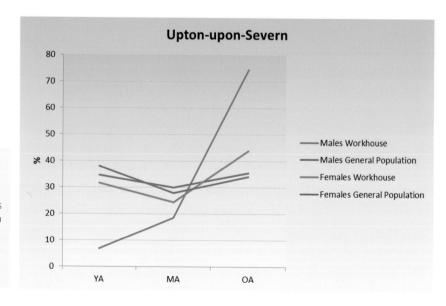

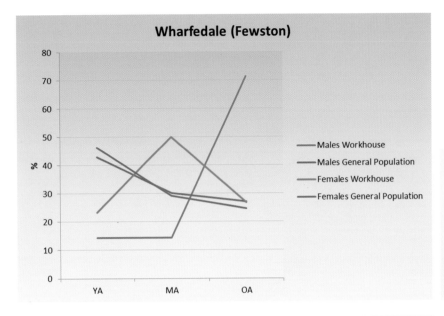

Figure 156 Age profile demographics comparing workhouse and general population from 1881 census data for Wharfedale (Fewston) (based on data from www.workhouses.org. uk) (YA = young adult, MA = middle adult and OA = old adult)

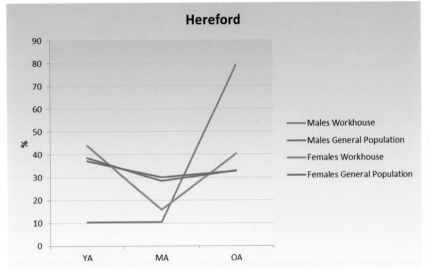

Figure 157 Age profile demographics comparing workhouse and general population from 1881 census data for Hereford (based on data from www.workhouses. org.uk) (YA = young adult, MA = middle adult and OA = old adult)

than in the general adult population. For male manual labourers, the period of their working life was linked to their physical capabilities. Unable to work in old age, many were not able to support themselves financially. Old age females, however, were probably less vulnerable to workhouse submission since they still had roles in child care, domestic service or being employed in less physically demanding crafts, such as box or hat making.

In comparison, in London, there were equal numbers of old males and old females

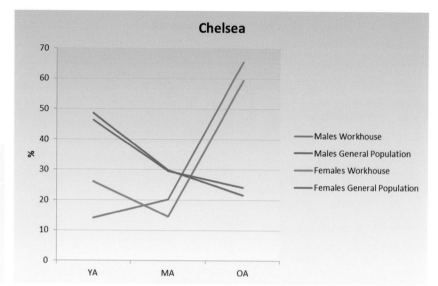

Figure 158 Age profile demographics comparing workhouse and general population from 1881 census data for Chelsea (based on data from www.workhouses. org.uk) (YA = young adult, MA = middle adult and OA = old adult)

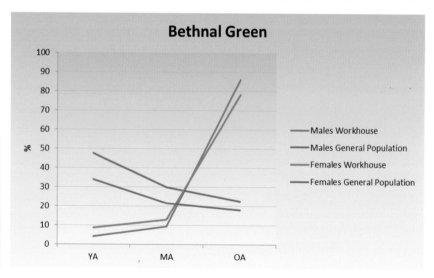

Figure 159 Age profile demographics comparing workhouse and general population from 1881 census data for Bethnal Green (based on data from www. workhouses.org.uk) (YA = young adult, MA = middle adult and OA = old adult)

in workhouse populations at Chelsea and Bethnal Green (Figs 158 and 159), with both present in relatively higher numbers than in the general adult population. Old aged females in London were as vulnerable as males and seemingly not incorporated into extended family roles, possibly as a result of increased migration rates into the City. This led to higher numbers of single status individuals and a subsequent lack of supporting family, especially in widowhood.

While physical fitness is a key factor, the perception of what people may consider to be the specific attributes of being older varies. Many of those living in the past may not even have known their exact chronological age, or have had, as we have in the present day, defined markers of having attained old age. Some people in the past may have felt older than they were if they were weak and frail, therefore believing themselves to be older than their chronological age. Others may have been perceived as older in relation to what they had achieved in life and some may even have added more years to their age to appear older in attempts of gaining esteem. The more common notions of what are seen as the marks of ageing are associated with diminished physical and mental functions of the body. The older person is viewed as not being so agile both physically and mentally, being more prone to chronic disease, mobility issues, impairment of hearing and vision and to the loss of elasticity to skin, causing wrinkles and sagging. It is these visual, cosmetic characteristics that are most readily identified as the representative image of an old aged person (Fig. 160). As Francesco Petrarca wrote in the mid-14th century, 'I admit that I am an old man. I read my years in my mirror, others read them on my brow.'

Throughout history, much emphasis has been placed upon the benefits of youth and striving to remain forever young. With the scrutiny more often placed on outward looks and particularly with pressure placed upon females, there have for many years been attempts to attain a constant youthful appearance. Much cost and effort is spent on trying to slow or reverse the signs of ageing with modifications ranging from weird cosmetic endeavours including snail secretions and cryogenic chambers, to multitudes of face creams, and the more extreme plastic surgery interventions. An article in Marketwatch in 2014, noted that 'our fear of wrinkles has manifested a global anti-ageing industry worth $261.9 billion'.

For the men and women in this study, the closest thing akin to a cosmetic

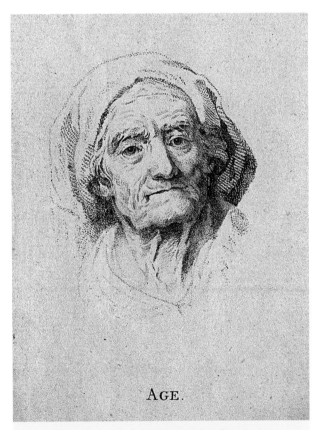

AGE.

Figure 160 Head of an old woman, Stipple engraving
(Wellcome Collection, cc-by/4.0)

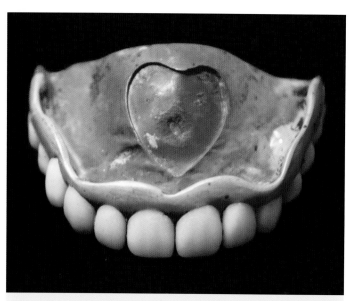

Figure 161 Set of 19th century vulcanite dentures with heart motif belonging to a female excavated from Swinton

(© Oxford Archaeology)

intervention may be seen in the examples of rather splendid dental interventions found with some of the Industrial era individuals. The loss of a person's teeth may be seen as an indicator of older age, with the effect of becoming edentulous or losing all the teeth, resulting in an almost sunken in appearance of the face. With the bone of the maxillae and mandible (upper and lower jaw) becoming resorbed and reduced in height, these changes cause a marked visual change to the face. Three females from the crypt at St Bride's Church, Fleet Street, London had bespoke handmade gold dentures for the maxillae (upper jaw) with gold poles and real teeth matched to compliment those they had remaining. Two individuals buried at Swinton had metal plates with porcelain teeth and one female a magnificent set of vulcanite dentures with resplendent teeth and a heart motif in the plate (Fig. 161).

Another attribute that would have affected the visual appearance and perception of an individual's age was the wearing of a wig. Following in the wake of royalty initially wearing wigs, they are more often associated as a mark of social status or learning but also provided a means for covering up baldness and the ravages of syphilis. They were particularly popular during the 17th and 18th centuries and the Georgian era is one where the visual image of gentlemen, who could have been both aristocratic or the self-made industrial elite, are frequently represented in paintings and pictorial representations of the day wearing powdered wigs, a man's wig known as a peruke or periwig (Fig. 162). Wig curlers have been found archaeologically and along the Thames foreshore (Fig. 163). A special tax on wig powder introduced by William Pitt in 1795 saw the eventual demise for wearing wigs by the end of the 18th century, although powdered wigs continue to be worn by English barristers in Court.

For those living in the Industrial era, particularly from the 1800s onwards, hygiene and beauty products became more accessible and affordable for the masses, with the development and formulation of well-known brands used for skincare to

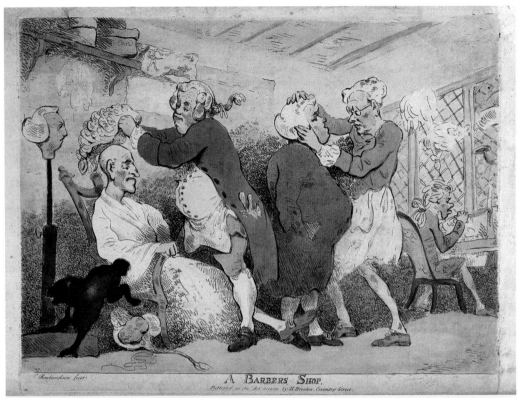

Figure 162 A barber's shop in which a fat barber places a wig on an old bald-headed man, an assistant barber who wears spectacles fits a wig on a stout man, in the right hand background a man sits on a chair facing a window, and in the left hand foreground a dog fouls a wig. Coloured etching after T. Rowlandson

(Wellcome Collection, cc-by/4.0)

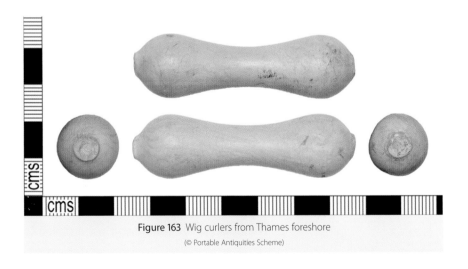

Figure 163 Wig curlers from Thames foreshore

(© Portable Antiquities Scheme)

ADVERTISEMENT.—Divinely beautiful are the effects produced by an incomparable Preparation recently discovered, combining the most exquisite and beautiful Cosmetics. Its radical purifying qualities render it infinitely superior to any Cosmetic ever known. By its unprecedented properties it removes freckles, pimples, spots, and all cutaneous eruptions; thus prevents those disorders which disorganise the beauty of the female countenance. In addition to the virtues of ROWLAND'S Kalydor already adverted to, it imparts a luxuriant and matchless beauty to the complexion, affords soothing relief to Ladies nursing their offspring; to Gentlemen after shaving, it allays the irritation and smarting pain, and renders the Skin smooth and pleasant. ROWLAND'S Kalydor will ever be found most efficient in its balsamic effects and delectable in its application.

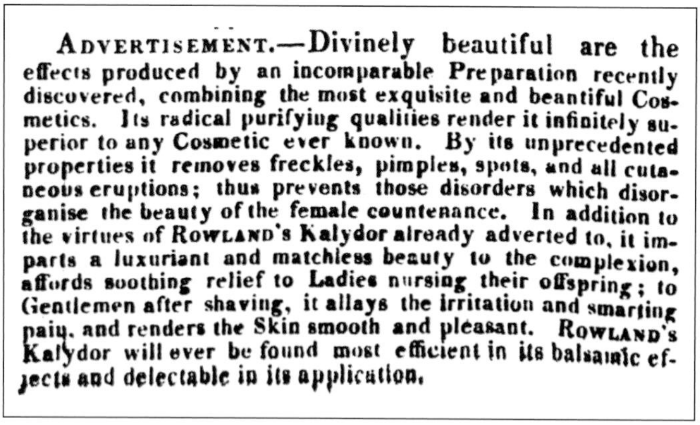

Figure 164 (left) Advertisement from the *Morning Post* newspaper, London Monday 14 June 1824. Newspaper image

Figure 165 (below) *Portrait of Elizabeth Vernon, Countess of Southampton, circa 1600*, artist unknown

try and diminish the signs of ageing. From the 18th century, the newspapers already had numerous advertisements, or 'puffs', to sell products that were ultimately a means to draw in individuals and focus on social identity (Fig. 164).

Whilst we cannot say directly from the analysis of the skeletal remains of the women and men in the study whether such products were utilised and applied, it could be suggested that those from both a high and low status background may have used animal fat based ointments. For those from a higher social status they may have gone further in transforming their appearance with the use of products to make their facial skin look paler and white, with the popular application of rouge to the cheeks and colouring of lips (Fig. 165).

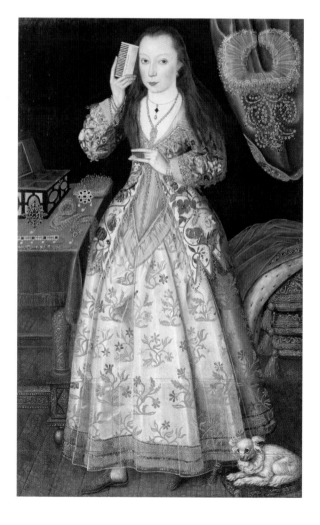

Age in the pre-Industrial period

The men and women from the pre-industrial era would have experienced a number of seismic shifts in working practices, economic and population fluctuations, all of which would have had implications for them reaching an older age. The evidence for social perceptions of old age in the pre-industrial era predominantly pertains to males, especially those of a higher social status, and relates mainly to civic duties. The 1285 *Statute of Westminster II* states that: 'A man may not be required to serve as a juror if he be in truth 70 years of age for that is the age prescribed by the Great Council as the limit of service'. The *Statute of Labourers* passed in 1349 refers to labourers and specifies the age of 60 as being the age at which certain physical tasks would be deemed no longer possible to carry out. Interestingly, this includes women as well as men. As Shulamith Shahar in 'Growing Old in the Middle Ages' identifies, there was no legal age for retirement or provision of pensions and fundamentally retirement from the occupation or role a person may have had depended, on a person's 'functioning abilities, economic and family circumstances, not on their chronological age'.

Estimates for life expectancy during this time are difficult to establish with availability of historical sources often limited and incomplete. Administrative records and wills, based predominantly on males, suggest that there was a relatively low life expectancy of only living into the 20s on average in the 11th and 12th centuries, which increased to the 30s but then had a steep decline during the impacts of the Great Famine and plague, increasing to the mid-30s later in the 14th and 15th centuries. It should also be considered that life expectancies during this time would be affected by fertility and infant mortality rates. Most historians agree, however, that living to older ages would have been commonplace. Chase, for example, refers to *The Differences in the Age of Man* by Henry Cuffe who, in 1607, divided old age into two chronological phases. The first, between the ages of 50 and 65, was marked by a 'will and readinesse to be doing'. The second, representing those aged 65 years and over, marked a considerable waning of the enthusiasm for 'doing' and is described as 'decrepit old age'. A similar attempt at charting old age is made by John Smith in 1666, which describes three stages of old age that progress from a 'crude' and 'green' state of still being able to go about business, to leaving off employments 'when God hath no work for them and they have no strength for him' and finally to being 'sickly decrepit and overgrown ... where their breath is corrupt, their daies are extinct and the grave is ready for them.'

A critical factor in the unpredictability of life expectancy during the pre-Industrial period were major climatic variations during the medieval period that affected food production, causing multiple episodes of famines within the UK, which was badly affected by the Great Famine (1315–1317) and pestilence affecting livestock (Great Bovine Pestilence 1319–1320). The outbreak in Europe of the Black Death (1347–1351), the pandemic plague caused by the bacteria *Yersinia pestis*, killed 25 million people and was first recorded in the UK in 1348, spreading rapidly throughout the country over the course of 2 years. It had a profound impact upon the UK rural and urban population, estimates indicating that at least a third of the population died from the disease, ultimately halting population growth for over 100 years. Excavations at Hereford Cathedral Close revealed a large pit with an estimated 300–400 bodies that had been dug to cope with the excessively high death rate. Ancient DNA analysis undertaken on skeletal remains from Hereford as well as at the Black Death burial ground at East Smithfield confirmed that the causative agent for the Black Death, *Yersinia pestis*, was present. The consequences of the disease were long lasting, which for many rural communities, in combination with the continued migration to urban centres, led to large numbers of villages ultimately becoming deserted. In pre-Industrial London, mass burials were also present at the burial ground of St Mary Spital, dating from 1120 to 1539. Although some of these pit burials dated to the time of the Black Death, many pre-dated and post-dated this plague outbreak. Instead, these were likely to have been associated with the well-documented periodic famines induced by climatic changes such as cooler temperatures, longer winters and wetter weather. As discovered by Don Walker (Museum of London Archaeology), a massive volcanic eruption in 1258 in the tropics, possibly in Mexico or Ecuador, led to a global 'dry fog' resulting in severe famines in England during the mid-13th century, at which time over half of the skeletal remains at St Mary Spital were buried in mass graves.

Age in the Industrial period

The period of the Industrial era and the concomitant effects of the Industrial Revolution saw major changes and upheavals to working ways of life, urban growth, environmental conditions and social divisions affecting life expectancy. With the advent of the Second Agriculture Revolution around 1700, there was an increase in the labour force and the implementation of more efficient methods of farming, enabling intensive arable cultivation to increase crop yields and to produce surplus that could then be sold on a commercial scale. The increasing food supply and agricultural productivity in Britain led to age expectancy starting to slowly increase along with population size. The famines that had markedly affected the pre-Industrial era were in decline but there were still many affected by hunger and malnutrition. Emma

Griffin notes that agricultural families in the late 18th and early 19th century spent 75% of their total weekly wages on food, 52.5% of wages being spent solely on bread. Any unexpected economic downturns, including poor harvests, had a profound effect on these low income families. Hunger and malnutrition still also prevailed in London. Despite earning more on average than their rural counterparts, City life encouraged criminal activity and drunkenness, leading to the failure of some 'breadwinners' to invest their higher earnings in food for the family. Social structure and employment status, therefore, had a substantial effect on health, ageing and the vulnerability of elderly dependents.

Edwin Chadwick's 1842 *Report on the Sanitary Condition of the Labouring Population of Great Britain* highlighted the striking differences in the life expectancy of the population based on occupation, social status and poverty, which eventually led to public health reforms. Chadwick claimed those living in the countryside lived longer than those in towns and his statistics for London showed the marked discrepancy for life expectancy between those of different social status (Table 17), with an average age of 43 years for the gentry or professional person compared to 22 years for the labouring classes across the whole of London. Occupation continued to define age and ageing, both in the physical and social spheres. Fitness for work continued to be the criteria used to define old age and by the 1840s, individual guilds would specify an age of expected 'retirement'. Karen Chase suggests that glassworkers might be expected to retire at 40 years old, carpenters at 50 and engineers at 55 years. Friendly societies in the mid- to late 19th century also often prescribed the age of 50 for which pensions could

Table 17 Average life expectancy from Edwin Chadwick's 1842 *Report on the Sanitary Condition of the Labouring Population of Great Britain*

Average age expectancy	Gentry/professional trades	Tradesmen	Labourers
Bethnal Green	45	26	16
Whitechapel	45	27	22
Kensington	44	29	26

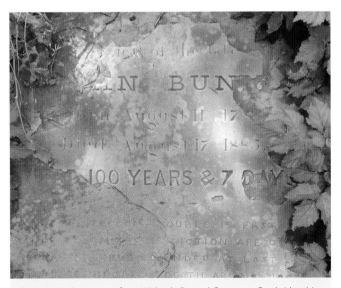

Figure 166 Gravestone from Wisbech General Cemetery, Cambridgeshire
(G. Western)

be drawn. In an essay entitled 'Who are the Old?' recalled by Chase, by 1881 the definitions of old age were extended so that a man between 40 and 50 was described as merely 'growing old' but that between 70 and 80 'he is aged'. Older than 80, and a man was 'venerable or patriarchal' but the ageing process all depended on the individual, whereby 'idiosyncrasy is everything'.

There is often the perception that people in the past did not generally reach particularly old ages, but the evidence shows that some people did indeed reach quite remarkable ages. For example, one gravestone dating to 1885 commemorates Mrs Ann Bunn (Fig. 166), who died at the grand old age of 100 years and 7 days.

The perhaps more intriguing lasting memorial to a person reaching a very considerable age is the wax effigy of Margery Scott (Fig. 167), who lived to be 108 years old. The wax model was made by the doll maker and wax modeller

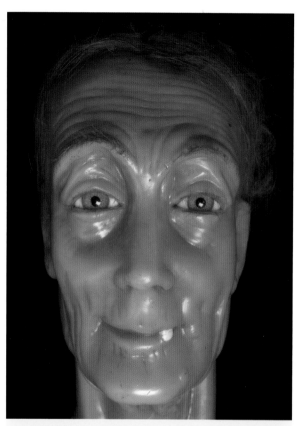

Figure 167 Wax model head of Margery Scott aged 108
(© Museum of London)

William Robins of London, in *c.* 1837. In contrast to the general impressions of life expectancy being shorter in the past, there are estimates of 8% living to be over 60 years old and there is clearly evidence that at least some individuals successfully made it into very old age, with even if commemorations to them were not particularly flattering.

Detecting age in the past

To investigate human longevity in the past, age at death estimates for the skeletal remains in this study were based upon standardised macroscopic ageing techniques as applied to the human skeleton in addition to any biographical data surviving from coffin plates. The macroscopic applications used for age estimation of adults are all related to processes fundamentally linked with degeneration. The methods for age estimation of the adult skeletal remains within the project used criteria following modern scientific standards based on dental wear, sternal rib ends and boney changes in the pelvis focusing on the areas of the pubic symphysis and auricular surface (Fig. 168). These joint surfaces located at the front and the back of the pelvis change form and degenerate as an individual ages, allowing age at death to be estimated by an examining osteologist.

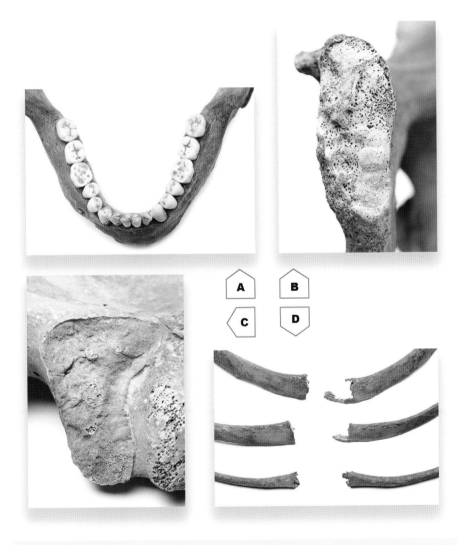

Figure 168 Areas of the skeleton used for age estimation in adults: (A) dental wear (mandible); (B) pubic symphysis (pelvis); (C) auricular surface (pelvis); (D) sternal rib ends (ossification of cartilage)
(© Museum of London)

However, with people all being individual, there is no precise uniformity to the ageing process in adulthood and so broad age categories are used, allowing for variance to be factored in. Individuals were identified as young adult (YA: 18–34 years), middle adult (MA: 35–49) and old adult (OA: 50+).

Where written evidence survives, such as burial records in parish registers and head stones, we can compare age profiles to those obtained from skeletal analysis. Data from skeletal remains from the Holy Trinity Church, as compared to contemporary

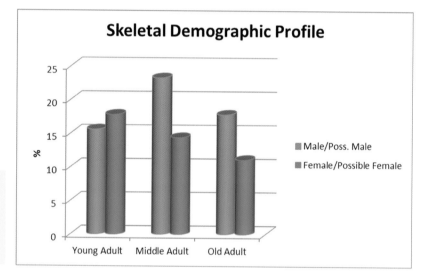

Figure 169 Demographic profile of the skeletal assemblage (young adult: 18–34 years, middle adult: 35–49 years and old adult: 50 years and over)

(Ossafreelance)

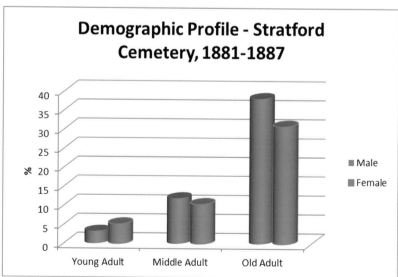

Figure 170 Demographic profile of Evesham Road Cemetery, Stratford-upon-Avon 1881–1887

(Ossafreelance)

burial registers from Evesham Road Cemetery, Stratford-upon-Avon indicate that there are fewer old age adults identified osteologically than are present in the burial records (Figs 169 and 170). This is a common issue in osteological studies caused by a lack of more accurate ageing techniques for archaeological skeletal remains.

No single source of data is entirely accurate for reconstructing age demographics in past populations and using skeletal data alone can be problematic. However, by combining and comparing as many different sources as possible, we are able to ascertain general trends that can give us an insight into how population dynamics have changed over time and how diseases of old age have changed in frequency. As part of this research project, demographic profiles of our study areas were compiled from both historic and skeletal sources where possible, to compare the numbers of people either living in London or outside the City who lived to old age, both in the pre-Industrial and Industrial periods to examine whether this changed over time. Migration away from rural to urban centres is a factor seen affecting demographics in the pre-Industrial and Industrial periods that must also be taken into account, with predominantly the young moving to seek work, causing an effect to the age profiles within the communities. While an influx of younger individuals will reduce the relative number of old age people in a community, out-migration of younger individuals will increase the relative number of old age people.

Archaeological demographic profiles

Using the age estimates from skeletal remains (Table 18; Figure 171) there was no significant difference in old age mortality outside of London between the pre-Industrial (32%) and Industrial periods (31.6%) and therefore old age mortality in the rural towns and villages remained relatively constant over time. However, old age mortality over the same period of time in London changed considerably, with significantly more old age adults present in the skeletal assemblages from the Industrial period (41.6% compared to 10.7%). The higher numbers of young adults in pre-Industrial London could be an indication of young migrants coming to London from rural locations, particularly in the wake of the devastating effects of the Black Death and famines. During the Industrial period, old age mortality in London was also higher than in rural towns and villages. Therefore, more old age people were present in the London Industrial sample than any of the others, a reflection perhaps of socio-economic changes with a growth of wealth and income, leading to improved living standards and increasing life expectancy for some.

Table 18 Archaeological Age profile for all age groups and periods

	Total sample	Young adults	Young adults %	Middle adults	Middle adults %	Old adults	Old adults %
Industrial London	799	256	32.0	211	26.4	332	41.6
Industrial non-metropolitan	526	191	36.3	169	32.1	166	31.6
Pre-Industrial London	456	254	55.7	153	33.6	49	10.7
Pre-Industrial non-metropolitan	572	224	39.2	165	28.8	183	32.0

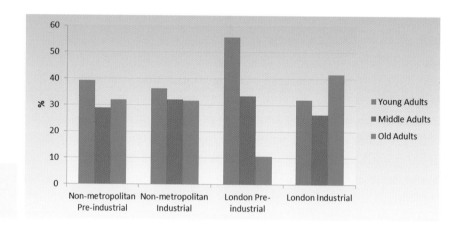

Figure 171
Archaeological
age profile

Historic age demographics

Bills of Mortality were the weekly statistics for recording burials in some London parishes undertaken between 1592 and 1858. As with all sources there can be limitations but analysis by Charlotte Roberts and Margaret Cox revealed an increase for life expectancy, which can be seen with the increase in old age adults from 45% of the adult population in the 1720s to 53.7% in the 1850s (Fig. 172).

The number of adults in their 50s was relatively stable throughout this time period but there were noticeable increases of those aged 60+ years, from 13.7% in the 1720s to 17.3% in the 1850s (Fig. 173). Numbers of those in their 70s similarly increased over the period. Using census data from the period 1851–1860, it is possible to reconstruct the age profile of living populations from both London and outside of the City (Fig. 174). In contrast to the archaeological data, significantly higher proportions of old age people (50+ years; 29.1%), including those that are 70+ years (6.4%), are found in towns and villages outside of London, where only 23.4% of the population were aged 50+ years and 4.0% over 70+ years.

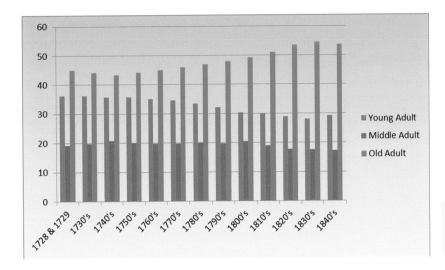

Figure 172 Age at death in London 1728–1850 for adults (after Roberts and Cox 2003)

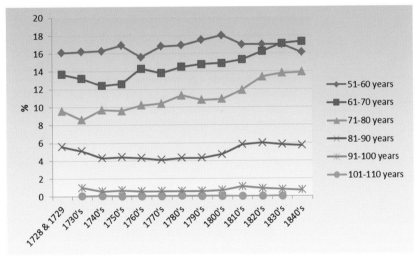

Figure 173 Percentages of old adults in decennial age groups (based on data from Roberts and Cox 2003)

The relative numbers of old age people at this time both in London and outside was much lower than in modern UK populations. Today, 38% of the adult population is aged 50+ years and 14.8% aged 70+ years. The proportion of 50+ years individuals, therefore, has grown by just over a third since 1851–1860 and that of 70+ years individuals has more than doubled.

From the 1851–1860 census data, those towns more involved in industry have the lowest proportions of old age individuals, possibly due to in-migration of younger individuals and as well as a lower life expectancy. Those towns whose economy is based on agriculture have the highest proportions of old age adults, possibly due to out-migration of young people to the towns and cities but also perhaps due to increased life expectancy in rural areas that Chadwick had reported around this time.

The 1851–1860 living population data compares well to the age profile obtained from contemporary mortality records (Fig. 175). Significantly higher proportions of individuals were dying in old age (50+ years) in rural towns and villages (57.1%) compared to London (47.9%), a pattern that was also seen into the 75+ years group (23.8% compared to 14.4%). However, in contrast to the living population, the type of economy was less of a factor. Although rural villages and towns tended to be the locations with higher rates of old age mortality, some towns more involved in industry had higher rates of old age mortality compared to some rural villages.

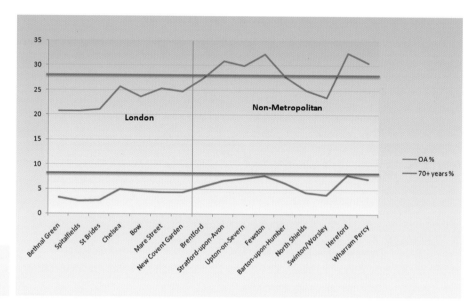

Figure 174 1851–1860 old age living population (Census data)

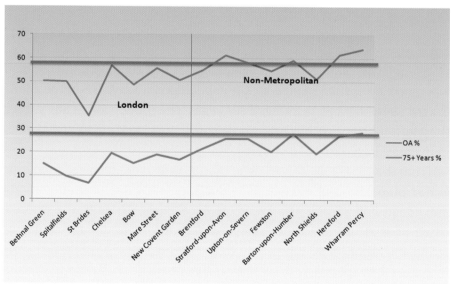

Figure 175 1851–60 old age mortality

Comparative modern mortality data from 2017 for England and Wales shows a mortality rate of 95.8% for those 50+ years and 68.9% for those 75+ years, indicating that the rates of old age mortality in modern populations are vastly higher than in the past, with increases on average of 36% higher for 50+ years and almost 50% higher for 75+ year olds.

In London, the skeletal data indicates that overall, areas of higher status had significantly higher rates of old age mortality (49.4%) compared to low status areas (36.6%), which in comparison had a significantly increased risk of death in middle age (31% v 18.4%) (Fig. 176).

This was also reflected by the 1851–1860 documentary mortality data (Fig. 177), though not to the same extent. This is explained by the fact that the documentary

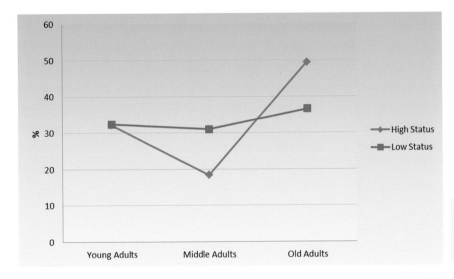

Figure 176 Comparison of high and low status adults from London Industrial skeletal populations

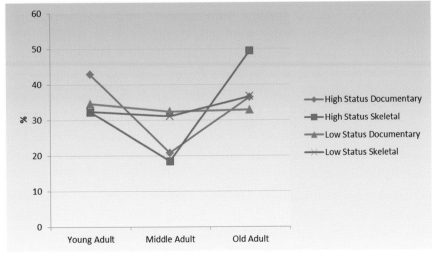

Figure 177 Comparison of high and low status skeletal data with documentary data

records cover a wider geographic area including individuals from higher and lower status residences, whereas our skeletal assemblages are more exclusive and consist of either high or low status individuals.

Overall, however, there were significant differences between the age profiles obtained using documentary information and ages from skeletal analysis. Old age people are under-represented in skeletal assessments (36.6%) compared to the 1851–1860 mortality data (52.5%). This means that although the skeletal remains identified as old age adults are likely to have been assigned to the correct age group, some old age individuals may have been misidentified as middle aged. The techniques used for the estimation of age for skeletal remains within archaeological collections are problematical and tend to underestimate the age of older individuals.

Conversely, in some high status skeletal assemblages, old age adults can be over-represented due to the social selection of older, more valued and affluent individuals according to funerary customs. Ages at death known from the biographical information of the higher status individuals from St Bride's crypt show that although the ages of the incumbents ranged from a few days old to 91 years, 61.5% were 50+ years old and 19.2% were 70 + years old. In other words, wealthy individuals may have not only been living longer but also attaining a higher social status as a corollary of being old aged. This may also contribute towards the discrepancy between the comparative numbers of old age individuals in our Industrial London skeletal population in relation to the historical data.

Changes in mortality age profiles over time

Looking at comparative rates of premature deaths (<75 years of age) is a means of assessing whether some populations have a lower proportion of people reaching old age than others. Using modern data from Public Health England in addition to mortality data from the 1851–1860 period, we can compare rates of premature deaths not only across different geographical locations but also over time. Comparing the rank of premature death prevalence amongst the study areas in our group, where our samples were ranked from 1 (lowest) to 14 (highest), it can be seen that the change in the relative number of premature deaths over time has varied widely in some areas (Fig. 178). Swinton, as part of Salford, still experiences one of the highest rates of premature deaths whereas central London, including the parish of St Bride's and Chelsea, have improved dramatically. The East End of London has seen little change and Bethnal Green, Bow and Spitalfields combined still has one of the highest rates of premature deaths in the group while Hackney (Mare Street) has relatively

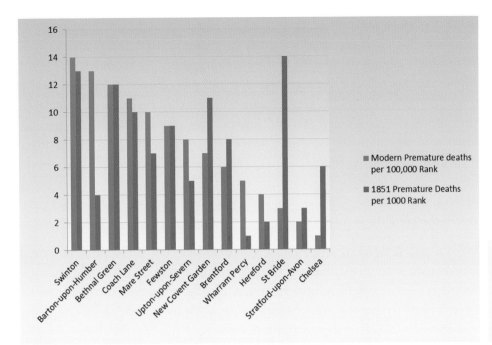

more premature deaths now than in 1851–1860, when it was a higher status area. Some towns located outside of London have experienced a similar relative increase in premature deaths, quite dramatically so, as in the case of Barton-upon-Humber, likely to be due to its continued urbanisation combined with its subsequent economic downfall.

Data from the *Statistical Digest of Rural England* (2018) indicates that over recent decades there has been a larger increase for average age at death in rural areas compared with urban areas, known as 'the greying of the countryside'. Our historic data would suggest that this trend for more old age adults present in rural communities has been present since at least 1851. Compared to the stable rates seen outside the City over time, our skeletal data appears to indicate that old age mortality is likely to have increased over time in London; however, we can see that social status in London had a significant effect on mortality profiles. This may reflect a wider trend for an increased life expectancy within wealthier populations in the Industrial period, as indicated by the historic surveys, but also could be influenced by the selection of older individuals in certain high status burial locations. The data from modern UK populations, however, confirms that economic prosperity is linked to increased life expectancy and lower rates of premature deaths.

Diseases of old age

With an increasingly ageing population in the UK today, there are seen to be inherent risks for higher disease burden and a greater demand placed upon social and health care structures. There is a much greater awareness today of diseases associated with getting older, which affect both the mental and physical health of people. Osteoarthritis and osteoporosis are two diseases which have become increasingly synonymous with the elderly.

Osteoarthritis: the clinical picture

Osteoarthritis is a degenerative musculoskeletal disorder that is the most common of the joint diseases, with an estimated 8,000,000 people in the UK affected (Arthritis UK). Its aetiology is still not fully understood. Anybody can develop osteoarthritis but older age is most frequently the primary cause, with wear and tear of the joints in combination with load bearing particularly affecting the hip and knee, smaller joints (hands and feet) and vertebrae (spine).

Factors to consider in relation to the disease are:

- The shape of the joint
- Developmental variations – e.g. dysplasia
- Living conditions
- Biomechanics
- Occupation
- Sex
- Muscles – strength and weakness
- Weight
- Genetics
- Ethnicity
- Underlying or secondary trauma
- Other joint disease

The foundation Arthritis Research UK and Imperial College London developed the Musculoskeletal (MSK) Calculator, a prevalence modelling tool for osteoarthritis of the hip and knee. They found that approximately 1 in 5 adults over 45 years in England have osteoarthritis of the knee and 1 in 9 adults of the hip.

Clinical research has shown that, overall, women have higher rates of osteoarthritis than men and also have higher rates of severe joint disease. The onset of osteoarthritis in men usually occurs before the age of 55, while for women it is over the age of 50, with suggestions of an association with the female menopause and a drop in the oestrogen hormone that helps to protect the cartilage from inflammation. Of the load bearing joints, the knee is the most frequently affected. Women are most often affected by knee arthritis: 19.7% of women compared to 16.6% men based on individuals aged over 45 years old (Public Health England, 2011–12).

The second most commonly affected joint is the hip. Although the average rate for hip osteoarthritis in adults aged over 45 years is lower for males (8%), than for females (13.6%), the hip is the most frequently affected joint in males. Physical and manual roles such as heavy lifting and load bearing have been linked to osteoarthritis of the hip while occupations involving kneeling and squatting have been linked with knee osteoarthritis. Recent legislation in relation to osteoarthritis as an occupational disease includes hip and knee osteoarthritis as an industrial injury, which could enable claims for compensation by workers in agriculture, coal mining, carpet fitting and farming.

Arthritis UK also identifies obesity as being an important factor in osteoarthritis, particularly of the knees, due to the increase in pressure on the joints. An obese person is 14 times more likely to develop knee osteoarthritis. Post-menopausal women have more fat around the stomach, placing greater pressure on the knees, which may in part be why more women have knee osteoarthritis. Across our study areas (Public Health England, 2011–12), the average rate of knee osteoarthritis in obese adults is 27% compared to 12.2% in adults of healthy weight. Similarly, a rate of 14.4% of hip osteoarthritis was found in obese adults compared to 8.4% in healthy weight adults.

Osteoarthritis in the past

In skeletal remains, the identification of osteoarthritis is made from the macroscopic changes visible in the bones and affecting the joint surfaces. Visual assessment of the actual bones and joint surfaces enables the processes of the breakdown of the joint to be seen, with the damage caused to the joint capsule and cartilage which provide the protective covering to the bones preventing friction between them. The onset changes may be classified as degenerative joint disease (DJD), a precursor to osteoarthritis, seen in the alteration to the joint surface with pitting and porosity, marginal osteophytic lipping (bony outgrowths) of the joint and ultimately eburnation (shiny surface), the pathognomonic (key) indicator of osteoarthritis. One older male adult from Chelsea Old Church aged 84 years at death, had bilateral osteoarthritis of the hips with the joint sockets for both sides showing breakdown

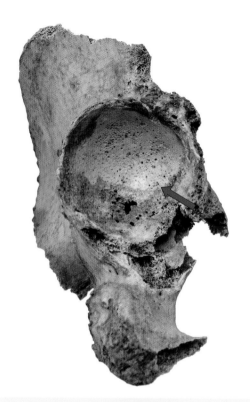
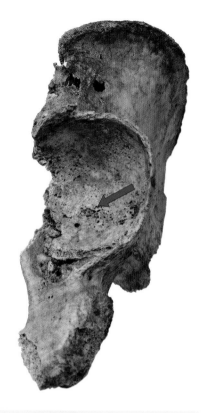

Figure 179 Bilateral osteoarthritis of the hips in an older male, Industrial London (OCU00 681) eburnation (red arrow) and macroporosity (blue arrow)
(© Museum of London)

of the joint surface (macroporosity) and eburnation (Fig. 179). Movement may have been painful and difficult but the very presence of the shiny eburnated surfaces of the hip joints are an indication of mobility with the action of the bones rubbing together producing the eburnation.

Knee OA

Rates of knee osteoarthritis (Fig. 180) were significantly higher in the rural villages and towns than in London in both the pre-Industrial and Industrial periods. In the Industrial period, the rate of knee osteoarthritis for the total population in areas outside London was 9.7%, much higher than the 3.5% present in the London population. The rate during the pre-Industrial period was 3.9% outside of London compared to 0.5% in the City (Table 19).

Rates of knee osteoarthritis increased over time both in London and in rural towns

Table 19 Knee osteoarthritis prevalence rates according to age and group in female (F) and male (M) adults according to age (YA = young adult, MA = middle adult and OA = old adult)

	FYA	FMA	FOA	MYA	MMA	MOA	Total
Knee osteoarthritis cases	2	4	17	0	2	14	39
Industrial London	196	138	241	124	164	256	1119
%	1	2.9	7.1	0	1.2	5.5	3.5
Knee osteoarthritis cases	4	4	16	0	7	16	47
Industrial non-metropolitan	85	77	62	77	111	72	484
%	4.7	5.2	25.8	0	6.3	22.2	9.7
Knee osteoarthritis cases	1	0	1	1	0	0	3
Pre-Industrial London	129	63	29	155	123	80	579
%	0.8	0	3.4	0.6	0	0	0.5
Knee osteoarthritis cases	0	3	7	0	2	2	14
Pre-Industrial non-metropolitan	64	58	39	57	92	53	363
%	0	5.2	17.9	0	2.2	3.8	3.9
Knee osteoarthritis cases	7	11	41	1	11	32	103
TOTAL	474	336	371	413	490	461	2545
%	1.5	3.3	11.1	0.2	2.2	6.9	4.0

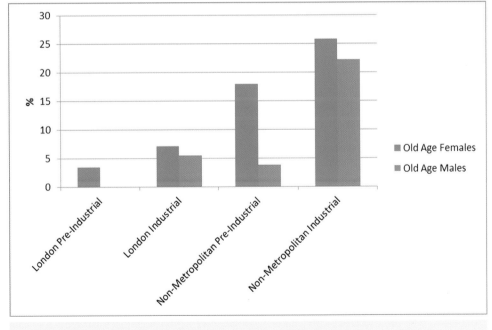

Figure 180 Percentage rates of knee osteoarthritis in old males and females for all periods

and villages and this increase was predominantly seen in old age males. This could be associated with an increase in their obesity levels over time or with changing occupations. In comparison, no significant differences in knee osteoarthritis were found in females over time.

Overall in London, there was no significant difference between rates of knee osteoarthritis in old age males and females in either the pre-Industrial or Industrial periods. In rural towns and villages, rates were higher in the pre-Industrial old age females compared to males but not during the Industrial period, when rates were similar between sexes. In London, there was no significant difference between rates of knee osteoarthritis in low or high status old age individuals, either male or female or of any age group.

Hip OA

Overall, significantly higher rates of hip osteoarthritis were consistently found in locations outside of London in both the Industrial (10.8% v 2.3%) and pre-Industrial (10.6% v 0.8%) periods, similar to knee osteoarthritis (Fig. 181). During the Industrial period, rates were only 3.5% in old age females and 5.8% in old age males in London compared to 20.8% and 30.2% outside of London. The same pattern was found in the pre-Industrial samples, where only 3% of old age females and 1.6% of males were affected by hip osteoarthritis in London compared to 30.6% of old age females and 19.2% of old age males outside the City (Table 20). Rates were consistently higher over time in those old age individuals living outside London. However, the overall rate of hip osteoarthritis significantly increased over time within London. No significant differences were present in rates of hip osteoarthritis between old age males and old age females in any of the groups and there was no significant difference in rates over time for either old age males or old age females in the City or in rural towns and villages.

In London, high status old age females were significantly less likely to have hip osteoarthritis (0.8%) compared to low status females (5.6%), although the same was not true of old age males, where status did not affect hip osteoarthritis rates. When looking at the frequency of hip osteoarthritis in the young and middle aged groups for high and low status individuals, there was no statistical significance.

Looking at a subsample of the London assemblage to see if there was a relationship between osteoarthritis and HFI or DISH, which are linked to being overweight, there was found to be no statistical significant relationship between them in old age adults. This may be an effect of the sample size, where the overall numbers of those individuals having HFI or DISH and osteoarthritis were small. It is also likely however, that individuals in the lower status assemblages developed osteoarthritis through the

Table 20 Hip osteoarthritis prevalence rates according to age and group in female (F) and male (M) adults according to age (YA = young adult, MA = middle adult and OA = old adult)

	FYA	FMA	FOA	MYA	MMA	MOA	Total
Hip osteoarthritis cases	2	0	9	0	1	16	28
Industrial London	204	144	260	133	182	278	1201
%	1	0	3.5	0	0.5	5.8	2.3
Hip osteoarthritis cases	4	4	15	0	12	26	61
Industrial non-metropolitan	98	85	72	90	136	86	567
%	4.1	4.7	20.8	0	8.8	30.2	10.8
Hip osteoarthritis cases	1	0	1	0	2	1	5
Pre-Industrial London	145	71	33	170	139	62	620
%	0.7	0	3	0	1.4	1.6	0.8
Hip osteoarthritis cases	2	6	15	0	11	14	48
Pre-Industrial non-metropolitan	71	74	49	68	117	73	452
%	2.8	8.1	30.6	0	9.4	19.2	10.6
Hip osteoarthritis cases	9	10	40	0	26	57	142
TOTAL	518	374	414	461	574	499	2840
%	1.7	2.7	9.7	0	4.5	11.4	5

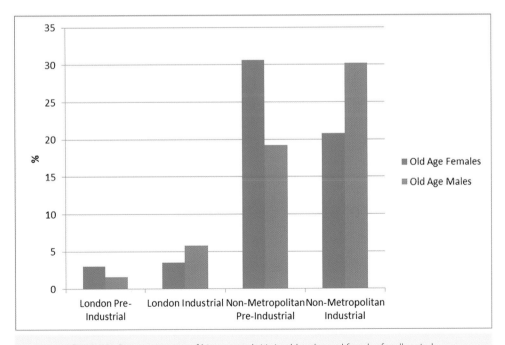

Figure 181 Percentage rates of hip osteoarthritis in old males and females for all periods

physical stresses of manual labour compared to high status people, who had higher rates of HFI or DISH associated with being overweight, but did not undertake manual labour. The role of manual labour as a key factor in the aetiology of osteoarthritis in the past in comparison to obesity is very likely to be the explanation for the higher rates of osteoarthritis in more rural locations compared to London and also the lack of significant difference in rates between males and females.

Osteoporosis: the clinical picture

Age UK indicate that within the current population of the United Kingdom there are almost 3,000,000 people estimated to have osteoporosis. It is a disease that is identified as the 'silent killer' with the symptoms often unknown until a person breaks a bone. Rates of osteoporosis appear to have increased in the modern era, raising the question as to why this may have happened and whether it is simply a consequence of an ageing population.

Osteoporosis is a metabolic disease affecting bone density and the ability of bone to remodel, making it more fragile and vulnerable to fracture. There are two types of osteoporosis: Type I and Type II. Type I is associated with post-menopausal women and Type II is identified as senile osteoporosis, affecting those over 70 years and higher numbers of females. It can also affect men, younger people, and those who have an underlying problem with bone density or suffering from other diseases such as cancer.

For the maintenance of bone remodelling two of the most important types of bone cells that work together in the formation of bone tissue are osteoblasts (bone forming) and osteoclast cells (bone resorbing). If there is an imbalance between bone formation and bone resorption, this then causes bone loss leading to osteopenia (minor bone loss) and ultimately osteoporosis. The causes of osteoporosis are multifactorial and the risk of developing it has been linked to:

- Sex – females and the menopause
- Age – over the age of 50 years
- Genetics/Family history – if members of family have suffered with osteoporosis related fractures
- Lifestyle – smoking, alcohol, lack of exercise, diet (lack of Vitamin D and calcium)
- Other diseases – e.g. cancer, rheumatoid arthritis
- Low body weight
- Medications

One in three women over the age of 50 and one in nine men in the UK suffers with osteoporosis. Many women going through the menopause will be prescribed

Hormone Replacement Therapy (HRT), which is thought to not only assist with the symptoms of menopause but can also help in the prevention of the loss of bone density. However, a study in 2002 made links between HRT and breast cancer, and subsequently the numbers of women undergoing HRT dropped rapidly from an estimated 6,000,000 in 2000 to an estimated 2,300,000 in 2017.

Osteoporotic fractures

The fractures most frequently associated with osteoporosis are in the vertebrae (spine), wrist (Colles fracture) and hip, the latter being used clinically as a means of calculating the clinical incidence of osteoporosis. In 2016 for England, Wales and Northern Ireland, the National Hip Fracture Database annual report (2017) recorded that over 65,000 people aged 60 or older presented to hospital with a hip fracture. The National Average for a hip fracture in 2015–2016 for adults over 65 years was 589 per 100,000 of the population (0.589%). The risk of hip fractures in the UK is almost four times higher for females compared to males, occurring on average at 77 years old. Those in their 50s have a 2% risk, with a marked increase to 25% for those in their 80s. The primary cause of hip fracture is a fall directly onto the hip joint. The elderly are particularly at risk if they are underweight or are infirm and prone to trips and falls from physical impairments and/or dementia.

The hip joint is made up of the pelvis and femur (thigh bone) and the classification of a hip fracture is made in assessing the specific area of the break and what type of break is present in the bone. Ninety percent of hip fractures consist of two main types:

- *Femoral neck fracture*: a fracture which occurs about 2.5–5 cm (1–2 in) from the hip joint (Fig. 182). A major complication of this type is that the blood supply to the femoral head may be severed causing bone death.
- *Intertrochanteric fracture*: a fracture which occurs 7.5–10 cm (3–4 in) from the hip joint (Fig. 183). Repair to this type of fracture can be easier as it does not interrupt the blood supply as can occur with the femoral neck fracture.

A study in 2010 by David Tanner and colleagues has shown that the types of hip fracture in men and women change differently with age and this differing pattern in the rates is believed to be a reflection of the type and rate of bone loss between the sexes. The most frequent type of fracture observed in women with increasing age was intertrochanteric fractures but for men with this type of fracture, the pattern was opposite. This indicates that for men and women the cause and prevention of the two types should be considered separately. Between 2003 and 2013, the proportion

Femoral Neck Fracture

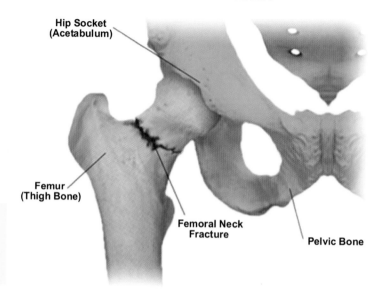

Hip Socket
(Acetabulum)

Femur
(Thigh Bone)

Femoral Neck
Fracture

Pelvic Bone

Figure 182
Femoral neck fracture

(© Stanford Health Care, https://
stanfordhealthcare.org/medical-
conditions/bones-joints-and-
muscles/hip-fracture/types.html)

Intertrochanteric Fracture

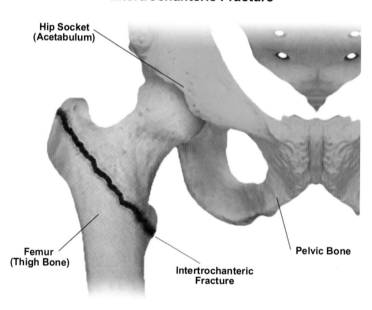

Hip Socket
(Acetabulum)

Femur
(Thigh Bone)

Intertrochanteric
Fracture

Pelvic Bone

Figure 183
Intertrochanteric fracture

(© Stanford Health Care, https://
stanfordhealthcare.org/medical-
conditions/bones-joints-and-
muscles/hip-fracture/types.html)

of men with hip fractures rose from 21.9% to 28.8%, with the incidence rate in older men (85 + years) having increased the most. One factor leading to this increase could be chemotherapy treatment for prostate cancer, which causes a drop in testosterone and a reduction in cortical bone density as a result.

Osteoporosis in the past
Bioarchaeological studies based on investigations of skeletal collections from the past have identified that osteoporosis has always been present, predominantly occurring in older females, as it does today. However, hip fractures in archaeological collections are not frequent (Table 21). As indicated by the historical data, a much smaller proportion of people in past populations lived into their 80s, who are the most commonly affected age group clinically. The overall rate of hip fractures in our study was very low; none were present in the pre-industrial populations and all occurred in the Industrial period (0.45%). Low status Bethnal Green had the highest number of cases, with six individuals affected.

Table 21 Hip fractures according to age and group in female (F) and male (M) adults according to age (YA = young adult, MA = middle adult and OA = old adult)

	FYA	FMA	FOA	MYA	MMA	MOA	Total
Hip Fracture Cases	1	0	3	0	1	4	9
Industrial London	204	144	260	133	182	278	1201
%	0.5	0	1.2	0	0.5	1.4	0.7
Hip Fracture Cases	0	1	0	0	0	2	3
Industrial non-metropolitan	98	85	72	85	131	86	557
%	0	1.2	0	0	0	2.3	0.5
Hip Fracture Cases	0	0	0	0	0	0	0
Pre-Industrial London	145	71	33	157	134	62	602
%	0	0	0	0	0	0	0
Hip Fracture Cases	0	0	0	0	0	0	0
Pre-Industrial non-metropolitan	71	74	49	68	117	73	452
%	0	0	0	0	0	0	0
Hip Fracture Cases	1	1	3	0	1	6	12
TOTAL	518	374	414	443	564	499	2812
%	0.2	0.3	0.7	0	0.2	1.2	0.4

Second metacarpal radiogrammetry
A more sensitive method for detecting osteoporosis in the past is based on radiogrammetry. This consists of metric analysis of the 2nd left metacarpal (fingerbone) to determine bone thickness, giving an indication as to whether the bone is healthy or whether any thinning has occurred.

Digital radiogrammetry was undertaken by measuring the total external width of the metacarpal (cortical width) and the medullary width (internal) at the mid-point of the bone (Fig. 184). These measurements are used to calculate the metacarpal index (MCI), which is the ratio of cortical thickness to the total bone width.

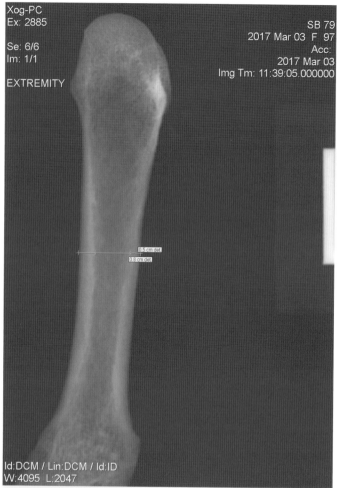

Figure 184 Left 2nd metacarpal showing the measurements for the Cortical Width (longer line, 0.8 cm) and the Medullary Width (shorter line, 0.5 cm) old adult female, Industrial London (SB79 97)

(© Museum of London)

A total sample of 1032 individuals, comprising young, middle and old male and female adults from each of the pre-Industrial and Industrial London and non-metropolitan groups were selected for radiogrammetry analysis. Only 2nd left metacarpals that were whole and well preserved were analysed. The samples were measured twice to ensure the data was consistent.

For defining those individuals with osteoporosis from the radiogrammetry results we followed two studies (Barnett and Nordin 1960; and Haara *et al.* 2006) based on large sample sizes that identified those individuals with a cortical index of <44 to be at increased risk of a hip fracture. In our study, individuals with an MCI score of <44 were, therefore, identified as osteoporotic.

As expected from the clinical information, the highest rates of osteoporotic low MCIs were in the old age adults and in particular old age females, who had consistently higher rates of osteoporosis than males across all the groups. For females and males, rates of osteoporosis generally increased with age (Figs 185 and 186). Additionally, females with hip fractures all had an MCI of <44. One male with a hip fracture similarly had a low MCI of <44 but unfortunately, we could not calculate the metacarpal index value for the other males with hip fractures in our sample.

Within our total sample of old age adults (Table 22), Londoners had the highest rates of osteoporosis in the Industrial period (21.8%) compared to the non-

Table 22 Males and Females in radiogrammetry sample with osteoporosis for all groups and periods in female (F) and male (M) adults according to age (YA = young adult, MA = middle adult and OA = old adult)

	FYA	FMA	FOA	MYA	MMA	MOA	Total
Low Cortical Index (osteoporosis)	4	6	34	4	1	8	57
Industrial London – radiogrammetry sample	85	48	92	69	62	101	457
%	4.7	12.5	37	5.8	1.6	7.9	12.5
Low Cortical Index (osteoporosis) cases	1	1	5	2	5	7	21
Industrial non-metropolitan – radiogrammetry sample	50	28	16	46	49	41	230
%	2	3.6	31.3	4.3	10.2	17.1	9.1
Low Cortical Index (osteoporosis) cases	6	5	5	8	3	3	30
Pre-Industrial London – radiogrammetry sample	40	15	12	51	27	28	173
%	15	33.3	41.7	15.7	11.1	10.7	17.3
Low Cortical Index (osteoporosis) cases	2	5	0	3	7	10	27
Pre-Industrial non-metropolitan – radiogrammetry sample	28	23	10	41	36	34	172
%	7.1	21.7	0	7.3	19.4	29.4	15.7
Low Cortical Index (OP)	13	17	44	17	16	28	135
Total	203	114	130	207	174	204	1032
%	6.4	14.9	33.8	8.2	9.2	13.7	13.1

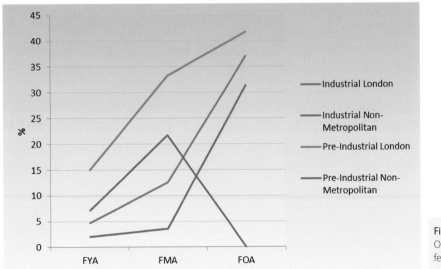

Figure 185
Osteoporosis in females

metropolitan areas (10.5 %). Londoners also had a higher rate in the pre-Industrial period (20%) in comparison to the pre-Industrial non-metropolitan older adults at (9.1%). This indicates that for both the Industrial and pre-Industrial period Londoners had significantly higher rates of osteoporosis.

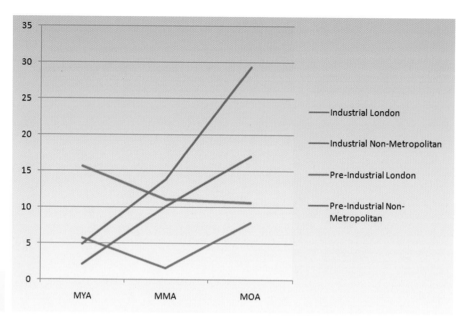

Figure 186
Osteoporosis in males

For London old age females, rates of osteoporosis remained consistent over time, with no significant differences in rates between the pre-Industrial and Industrial period for either group (Table 22). There were, however, significantly lower rates of osteoporosis for older males outside London in the Industrial period (17.1%) compared to the pre-Industrial period (29.4%). Additionally, in the Industrial period, there were no significant differences between rates of osteoporosis between low and high status individuals in London of either sex or in any age group.

It was not possible to compare fairly our female non-metropolitan pre-Industrial sample to any of the other groups because this sample was too small. However, old age males outside of London in the pre-Industrial period had a significantly higher rate of osteoporosis (29.4%) than their contemporaries in London (10.7%), a pattern that was repeated in the Industrial period (17.1% v 7.9%).

What is perhaps surprising are the relatively high rates of osteoporosis that were found in younger and middle aged adults in the pre-Industrial period, which would not be expected today. In fact, there was no significant difference in the rates of osteoporosis in either males or females between the young, middle or old age groups in pre-Industrial London. Looking more closely at the data from St Mary Spital and comparing the famine-related mass burial pits to the rest of the burials (Fig. 187), there was no significant difference between the rates of osteoporosis in each sample (Mass burial pits = 23.1%, other burials =13.1%). However, despite there being no difference in age profiles between the burial types, the age profiles of those

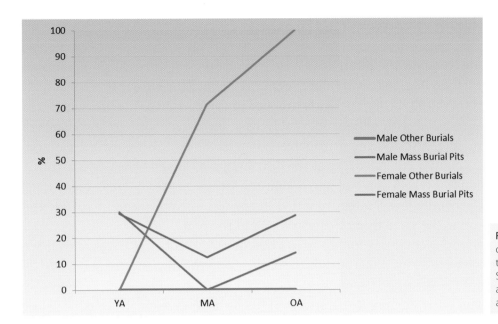

Figure 187 Rates of osteoporosis in the burials from St Mary Spital according to age and burial type

individuals with osteoporosis did differ between the burial types. In the mass burials, osteoporosis was found in significantly more young female and male adults (29.6%).

The higher rates of osteoporosis in these young adults at St Mary Spital could have been caused by periods of malnourishment and famine. Medical studies based on examination of animal models, individuals who have lived through times of famine from periods of conflicts, Holocaust survivors and those with eating disorders, all show a connection between starvation and osteoporosis incidence, in some cases premature and resulting from malnutrition *in utero* (i.e. maternal nutritional deficiency and fetal programming of physiological parameters) or in early childhood. The higher rates of osteoporosis in young and middle aged adults in the wider pre-Industrial populations found here, corroborating earlier research undertaken at Wharram Percy by Simon Mays (English Heritage), could similarly be related to malnutrition and famine events. This evidence for the combination of reduced longevity and increased premature ageing in the pre-industrial period lends support to the 'thrifty telomere' hypothesis proposed by D. T. Eisenberg. He suggests that the shortening of telomeres (the caps at the ends of chromosomes protecting DNA molecules) that occurs in early life in response to physiological stress (i.e. famine) as an energy saving mechanism, preventing energy-expensive cell proliferation, contributes to premature ageing and death.

Age-related diseases: the present

The general trend for the future is that the population will increasingly become an older population (Fig. 188), with more people living into the old age bracket despite life expectancy itself having currently dropped in comparison to the previous years. Diseases associated with old age inevitably have increased, with greater numbers affected by osteoarthritis and osteoporosis than in the past, with distinct patterns across the country. When looking at the distribution of hip and knee osteoarthritis for individuals over 45 years of age within the UK in our study areas today (Figs 189–192), generally lower rates are found in London in comparison to outside the City, mirroring the same trend that was found in the past.

The national average rate for hip osteoarthritis in 2011–2012 was 10.9%; rates above the average were all locations outside of London, with the higher rates in Calderdale (Fewston) at 11.6%, Salford (Swinton) at 11.7%, NE Lincolnshire (Barton-upon-Humber) at 11.3% and Herefordshire (Hereford) at 11%. The London boroughs were all below the national average with the lowest rate in West London (Kensington and Chelsea) at 9.6%. The overall modern rates of hip osteoarthritis are approximately the same now as found in the past in our non-metropolitan populations. A similar geographic distribution of hip osteoarthritis was found for both males and females. The national average for males is currently 8% and for females 13.6%. The highest rates for both males (8.7%) and females (14.6%) were from Salford (Swinton). The lowest rates again for the males and females were from West London (Kensington and Chelsea) with males at 6.9% and females at 11.9%.

A comparable pattern was seen with knee osteoarthritis, where the areas above the national average (18.2%) were all outside London, with the highest rate in Calderdale (Fewston) at 19.2% and the lowest rate in West London

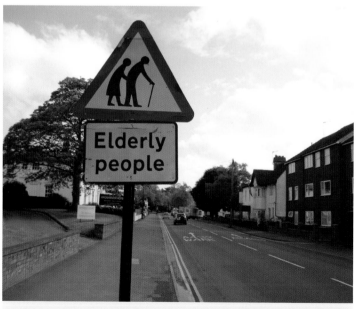

Figure 188 Road sign to alert for elderly people crossing
(A J Leon, cc-by/2.0, https://www.flickr.com/photos/ajleon/4662995633)

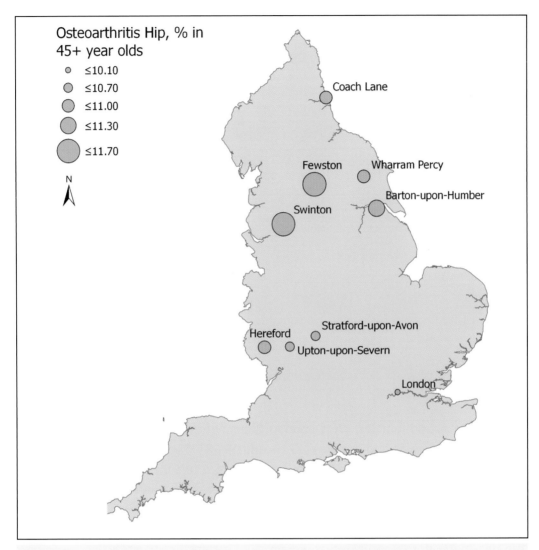

Figure 189 National statistics for osteoarthritis of the hips percentage in 45+ year olds (Public Health England, 2011–12)

(Kensington and Chelsea) at 14.6%. The national average prevalence rate was higher for females at 19.7% compared to males at 16.6%; the highest rates again were outside of London. For males, the highest rates were in Salford (Swinton) at 18.2% followed by NE Lincolnshire (Barton-upon-Humber) at 17.7%, and Calderdale (Fewston) at 17.5%. Female rates for knee osteoarthritis followed a similar pattern with the highest rates in Salford (Swinton) at 21.6%, NE Lincolnshire (Barton-upon-Humber) at 21.1% and Calderdale (Fewston) at 20.7%. In comparison for London, the rates for males and females with knee osteoarthritis was lower overall and below the national average

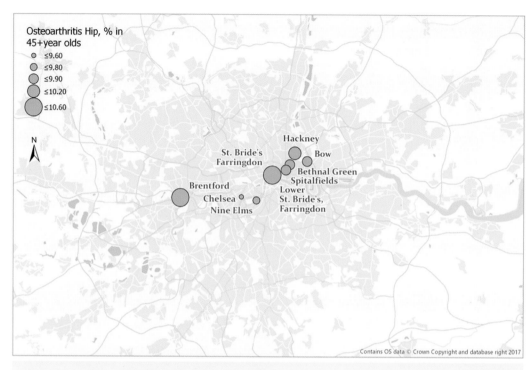

Figure 190 London statistics for osteoarthritis of the hips percentage in 45+ year olds (Public Health England, 2011–12)

for both males and females. West London (Kensington and Chelsea) again had the lowest rates for males and females (13.1% and 15.9%). The highest rates in London were in Hounslow (Brentford) at 17.5% for males and 19% for females.

The rates of knee osteoarthritis overall are much higher now than we found in this study in past populations and is most probably due to the increase of individuals excess weight. Those locations with high rates of osteoarthritis of the hip and knee also had high rates of adult excess weight. NE Lincolnshire (Barton-upon-Humber) and Salford (Swinton) had the highest rates of excess weight for adults at 69.7% and 67.1% respectively, and Calderdale (Fewston) at 64.5% only marginally below the national average (64.8%). In contrast, all of the London areas had the lower rates of osteoarthritis, with the lowest in West London (Kensington and Chelsea) at 47.3%, followed by the Tower Hamlet areas at 52.5%. Hounslow (Brentford) was the area with the highest London rate for excess weight at 62.7%, which also had the highest London rates for knee osteoarthritis.

Osteoporosis prevalence rates followed a similar pattern to those of osteoarthritis. Higher rates of osteoporosis were predominantly outside London and lower rates in the London areas. (Figs 193 and 194). With the rates for osteoporosis being based on

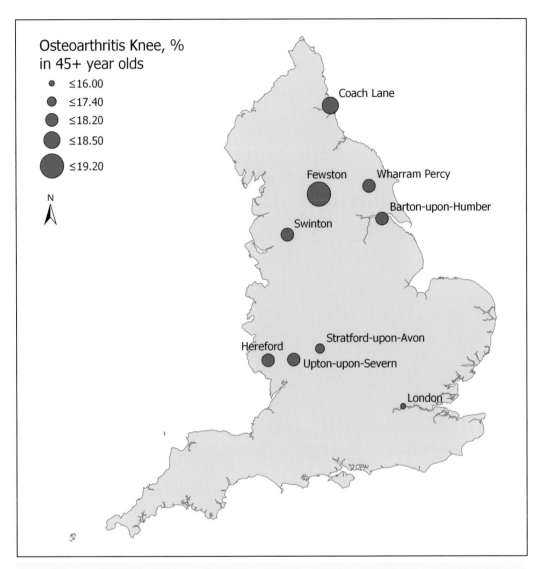

Figure 191 National statistics for osteoarthritis of the knee percentage in 45+ year olds (Public Health England, 2011–12)

hip fractures, the national average for 2015/16 for admission to hospital with a hip fracture was 589 per 100,000 for those 65+ years old. The London areas of West London (Kensington and Chelsea), and Central London (St Bride's and Lower Churchyard, St Bride's Farringdon Street) had the lowest rates at 391 and 400. Outside of London, Upton-upon-Severn (Worcester) had the lowest incidence rate at 506 and the highest at 722 was in NE Lincolnshire (Barton-upon Humber). The areas of London with above average rates were in Tower Hamlets (Bow, Spitalfields and Bethnal Green) at 671.

The osteoporotic hip fracture rate for females in all of the areas was higher when

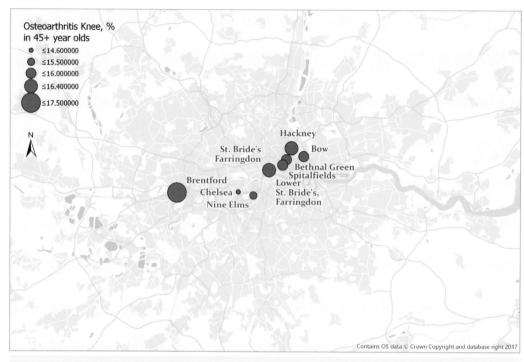

Figure 192 London statistics for osteoarthritis of the knee percentage in 45+ year olds (Public Health England, 2011–12)

compared to males (65+ years). Outside of London, the highest rate for females was in North Tyneside (Coach Lane) at 850 per 100,000, above the national average of 710. The highest rate for males was in NE Lincolnshire (Barton-upon Humber) at 520, above the national average of 416. For females and males in the London areas, the lowest rates were in Central London (St Bride's and Lower Churchyard, St Bride's Farringdon Street), at 439 for females and 348 for males. The highest rates for males and females were from London in the Tower Hamlets (Bow, Spitalfields and Bethnal Green) at 572 for males and 735 for females, which were the highest rates overall for London.

Comparing males and females, there is a moderate correlation between rates of osteoporotic hip fractures according to location but there are also clearly some differences between the sexes (Figs 195 and 196). Between 2015 and 2016, higher rates for males tended to be in low status areas of London compared to the lower rates in high status areas of the City, with the towns outside of London having rates in between these two extremes. Hip fractures in females were not so uniformly distributed across the City or between the City and outside of it, indicating that neither social status nor location was as influential. For females, age was the key factor in sustaining a hip fracture.

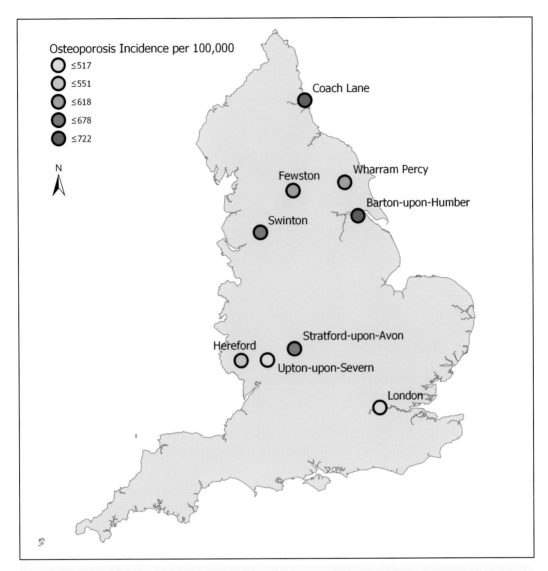

Figure 193 National statistics for osteoporosis incidence in the UK (Public Health England 2015–16)

As in the past, malnutrition is a factor to consider in the prevalence of osteoporotic hip fractures and may be one of the underlying causes of higher rates in males from low status areas. Older patients admitted to hospital with a hip fracture may suffer from the effects of being undernourished and overall, it is recorded that up to a third of patients having suffered from a hip fracture will die in relation to their age and fragility, partly caused by malnutrition. The relationship, between osteoporotic hip fractures and nutrition remains an area of continued debate. Further studies are

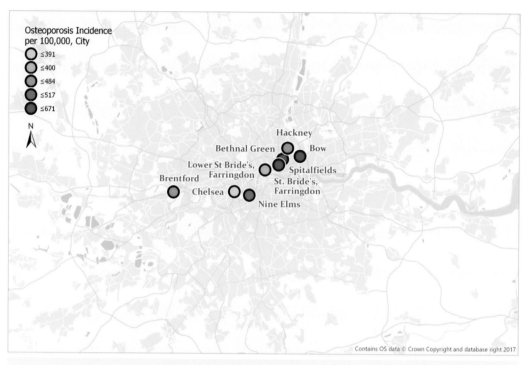

Figure 194 London statistics for osteoporosis incidence in London (Public Health England 2015–16)

needed due to the inconsistencies in assessing malnutrition in different hospitals, producing wide-ranging and not necessarily reliable results. In the UK in 2016, the cost to the NHS and social care was £1 billion with treatments and care needed for supporting those people having suffered from such a fracture.

Although more commonly being diseases attributed to old age today our data indicate that, in the past, factors other than old age and obesity, such as occupation and malnutrition, were previously as important in the causation of these conditions. As such, many people from the pre-Industrial period experienced accelerated or premature ageing compared to today due to periods of starvation, malnourishment and to intensive manual labour. Though this continued to an extent in the Industrial period, the ageing process started to differ, especially in high status individuals in London, with a reduction of osteoarthritis and osteoporosis in middle age accompanied by increased longevity, corresponding to increases in food availability. Famine-related osteoporosis, for example, was not present even in the low status individuals in industrial London. As longevity has continued to increase and our living environments have continued to change, so have the patterns of ageing, with rates of osteoporosis-related hip fractures increasing due to higher numbers of

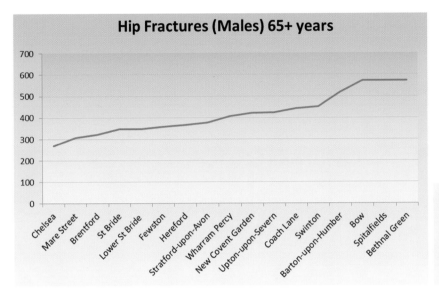

Figure 195 Age-sex standardised rate of emergency admissions for fractured neck of femur in males aged 65+ per 100,000 population (Public Health England 2015–16)

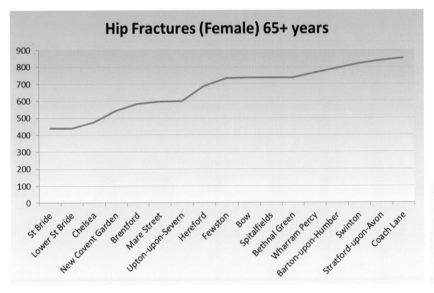

Figure 196 Age-sex standardised rate of emergency admissions for fractured neck of femur in females aged 65+ per 100,000 population (Public Health England 2015–16)

adults 80+ years surviving. Osteoarthritis rates have also increased over time as well due to obesity in older age rather than physical stresses. The rate of hip fractures of 0.34% in the Industrial period of those aged 50+ years compared with the modern rate of 0.589%, based on those aged 65+ years, shows that as the population has aged, the rate of hip fractures has almost doubled, reflecting the general trends seen in increasing rates of age-related disease prevalence today. What is also clear is that past and present, there are often significant geographical differences in rates of ageing and age-related diseases closely linked to variation in lifestyle and economic status.

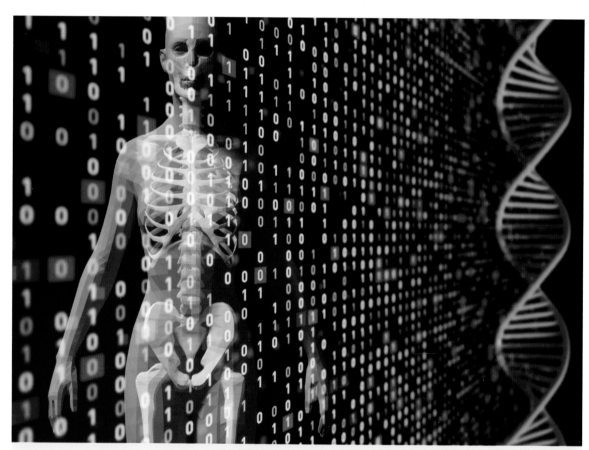

Figure 197 *The Human Engine*

(Shutterstock.com)

Conclusion:
The human engine

It is no exaggeration to say that, for the most part, the industrialisation of the City has been a grotesque assault on the health of Londoners. However, this was not a uniform process across all areas and all communities. From the 11th century, London grew from a walled town of the traditional Square Mile (2.9 km²), functioning as a high status port and royal administrative centre surrounded by villages and country estates, to an area now covering 608 square miles (1575 km²) of brick, stone, glass, steel and tarmac enclosing small areas of parkland, the 'lungs of London', as Charles Dickens referred to them in 1839. The archaeology of human remains from London in its nationwide context demonstrates how the diverse range of living and occupational environments in the City has been a key factor in disease patterns in the past, prompting a trend that has continued into the present day. In its prevailing working ethos of need, speed and greed, London in the Industrial period systematically divided its citizens according to their age, sex and social class, dictating in robust terms what jobs people did, how long they worked, the sort of housing they lived in, the sort of food they ate and ultimately, how long they lived. Though some generalised health effects were specific to London's unique status as the most densely populated metropolis in the world, with no-one escaping its all-encompassing choked-up and smoke-filled turbulent streets, the social engineering of the City's inhabitants became critical to Londoners' health outcomes. Over time, some of the adverse effects of industrialisation have been reversed by new safety legislation, medical advances and technological developments spurred on in the pursuit of civic progress, or by changing tastes of conspicuous consumption. However, others have continued, and of even more concern are new and emerging disease patterns in the City only rarely encountered in the past. The tangible evidence provided by this research, which could only have been achieved through the osteoarchaeological study of human remains using the latest imaging technologies, repeatedly highlights the importance of the local environment, and ultimately, the social status that goes hand in hand with it, for an individual's health and life expectancy, both in the past and the present.

Trauma

Accidents have been a part of the human condition throughout time and for the most part, have actually been more frequent outside of the City in rural areas dependent on agriculture. However, industrialisation reversed this trend and rates of fractures, particularly of the ribs, hands and lower arms, increased in London due to the boom of manufacturing in the City and its increased reliance upon physical manual labour. In contrast, risk of fracture decreased slightly outside the City. Males of low status were the most at risk of trauma in London and this risk appears to have continued into old age, a trend also seen in low status females. The higher risk of males to trauma in the City, which is still seen today, was due to gender-specific job roles exposing low status males to higher risk manufacturing occupations, in unregulated working environments that often included institutionalised drinking on the job. Although occupationally related deaths and accidents have been dramatically reduced due to health and safety rules, older males are still at the highest risk of death in the work-place, making the recent shift towards raising the age of retirement questionable. This has become less of an issue for London compared to other towns, however, due to its return to more office-based vocations. Road traffic accidents seemingly have been a threat since the invention of the wheel and today are most frequent outside of City with the exception of Inner London itself, which experiences rates of road deaths far higher than the national average. Interpersonal violence was also a persistent issue with high rates of violent deaths seen in the most densely occupied and poorest areas throughout Britain. Though the limited skeletal evidence for sharp force trauma was fairly low in all locations, knife crime today is now significantly more frequent in London.

Air pollution

Our study has produced clear evidence from the analysis of the human skeletal remains of Londoners that air pollution during the Industrial period, encompassing atmospheric pollutants, occupational dust and contagious lung diseases, posed a dramatically higher risk to health compared to areas outside the City. An unprecedented 19.5% of Londoners suffered from chronic inflammatory lung disease, though this was mitigated by social status and biological sex. Over 25% of low status individuals suffered chronic pulmonary inflammation, compared to only 9% of high status individuals. The vast majority of these low status males were part of an exploited workforce, some of whom were single migrants, exposed to extraordinarily poor working conditions involving occupational dust, ill ventilated work-spaces, smoke filled pubs and cramped, overcrowded, poor quality living accommodation. Air pollution in the City was superabundant compared to the rural towns and villages included in this study, where even during the Industrial period rates of chronic lung inflammation were only 4.2%. Several measures have been introduced to combat air pollution in the City and rates of occupational lung diseases such as pneumoconiosis are much reduced as a result of workplace regulations. However, occupational asthma and lung cancers arising from a new suite of occupational respiratory pollutants arising from the digital revolution, biotechnology and food processing are a growing health concern, particularly amongst an ageing workforce.

Cancer

It is difficult to compare directly rates of cancer over time because of how our understanding and recognition of cancer has evolved. Diagnostic and statistical criteria have changed as our medical knowledge has progressed and so historical medical records of cancer are not very helpful in understanding whether the number of cancer cases has increased over time. However, the radiographic survey undertaken here to identify cases of metastatic bone disease and multiple myeloma in the past revealed that these two conditions occurred at a much lower rate and appear to have increased over time. It is not clear whether the same can be said for all cancers that did not affect the skeleton, however. Most cases in our sample occurred in the Industrial London population, though overall the numbers of metastatic bone disease and multiple myeloma cases were very low. Today's cancer mortality statistics highlight London as a hotspot. The cause of the recent increase in cancer deaths is complex. Several of the areas both in and outside of London with high cancer mortality rates experience high population density and also have high levels of socioeconomic deprivation. Socioeconomic deprivation not only is often associated with lower uptake of cancer screening programmes but also with many lifestyle factors that put people at higher risk of developing cancer, such as smoking, being physically inactive, poor diet and obesity. Specific cancers, such as lung cancer, for example, can vary geographically according to local rates of smoking and obesity rather than according to the location of cancer cases in or outside of London. Population density, local variation in lifestyle factors as well as health service funding and delivery all have significant impacts on cancer outcomes. Cancer rates continue to increase today but so do positive outcomes following treatment.

Obesity and metabolic syndrome

Obesity is a problem of many consequences, not least of which are cancer and type 2 diabetes, which in modern populations are becoming increasingly common. It is not possible to calculate directly weight from the human skeleton but two skeletal conditions that are likely to be related to obesity and metabolic syndrome can be used to gain some insight into obesity in the past. Looking at rates of Diffuse Idiopathic Skeletal Hyperostosis (DISH) in older males and Hyperostosis Frontalis Interna (HFI) in older females, an increase over time in both these conditions was detected. Furthermore, both these conditions were considerably more frequent in males and females of higher social status in London, indicating that wealthier citizens were the most likely to be overweight or obese from a lack of physical exercise and the overconsumption of extravagant foodstuffs. Historically, the hectic nature of the busy London environment with its cosmopolitan mix of tenants, visitors and migrant labourers has created a constant market for ready-made food. This varied considerably in quality and for some was the only source of cooked meat. Females also started to frequent eateries and confectioners, selling pastries based on the latest fashionable food import, sugar. The rising demand for sugar over the 18th and 19th centuries eventually made it a common commodity and led to its decline in popularity with the upper classes. Instead, it became a necessary source of calories for low status workers and also a cheap preservative in the form of jam. Unlike HFI, a higher rate of dental caries resulting from sugar consumption was present in low status females, who although consuming more sugar, would have been much less likely to have been overweight or obese than high status women due their physical workload. In today's population, excess weight, dietary standards and physical inactivity are all closely linked to economic deprivation, a reversal of the trend seen in the industrial past. Obesity is currently an epidemic affecting the majority of adults in the UK today because of our continued hectic lifestyles, sedentary jobs and obsession with packaged, convenience foods containing saturated fats like palm oil as preservatives.

Ageing and age related diseases

Our investigations into the ageing process through time highlight that this was far from a predictable, uniform experience. The process of growing old has changed. The pre-Industrial period saw waves of poor harvests, famines and epidemics that had profound and long-term changes on the population. Overall, the age demographic for areas outside of London remained reasonably constant, with approximately a third of individuals in our sample dying in old age in both the pre-Industrial and Industrial eras. However, the pre-Industrial populations were ageing prematurely, most likely as a result of poor *in utero* and childhood nutrition caused by intermittent periods of hunger, as demonstrated by the higher presence of osteoporosis in young adults buried in famine-related mass burials. In addition, pre-Industrial rural populations experienced considerably higher rates of joint degeneration in middle age. By the Industrial period, food production had vastly increased, and though food was still not plentiful for all, its supply was apparently sufficient overall to cause a drop in osteoporosis in young and middle aged adults, so that its aetiology in the Industrial period began to resemble what we see today, significantly increasing in old age and especially affecting females. Osteoarthritis, however, showed little abatement or even increased for some living outside the City throughout the Industrial period. To some extent, this may reflect the increased numbers of old people seen in 19th century historic records in rural towns and villages compared to London. Overall, however, the data indicates that until technology took over as the main means of manufacturing and agricultural practice in the mid-20th century, the manual labour still required had a significant impact on rates of joint disease and was a key factor in its causation, in addition to age. Londoners, by comparison, experienced relatively little osteoarthritis, even in old age, despite comparable rates of osteoporosis. In the pre-Industrial period, the higher number of London's high status citizens along with the higher proportion of clerical roles has reduced overall rates of joint disease. Later, we begin to see the effects of industrialisation in creating a larger, intensively labouring lower class alongside a larger, non-labouring middle class. Rates of osteoarthritis increase and high status skeletal assemblages consisted of more individuals dying in old age, possibly having achieved a higher status in their social circle by living longer. Osteoarthritis is present in higher rates today due to increased numbers of old age adults as well as increased levels of obesity, though occupation is still a recognised risk factor. Osteoporotic hip fractures, however, were still quite rare until there were significant increases in the number of those living into very old age, as has been seen since the mid-1970s.

Comparing the skeletal remains of London's labourers, domestic servants, craftsmen and socialites to those of the farmers, fishermen, housekeepers and market traders from rural towns and villages lucidly illustrates how the human body has been ravaged by the various noxious afflictions we have created in our living environments, largely through our own agency. This is never more evident than through the Industrial period, where bodies have been pushed to physical extremes, often fatally so, in pursuit of financial gain, profit and status. In the pre-Industrial period, the human body experienced accelerated ageing from a reliance on harvests that were susceptible to failures and from the intensive manual labour required: however, while the UK was still largely agrarian, this was more equally experienced between adults, male or female. In contrast, the hierarchical social structure that industrialisation inherently commands has permeated all the aspects of health we have examined here from its inception. We see the hallmarks of proto-modern health patterns emerging amongst the high status London urbanites, whom experienced increased longevity and age-related diseases, probably along with increased obesity and related metabolic diseases, while low status groups continue to bear the burden of respiratory diseases, occupational trauma and premature degenerative diseases. This is a continuing theme in our current age of technological reliance and consumerism, even though medical advances and improved living environments have, until recently, helped more of us to live longer than ever before. However, our recent victorious longevity may prove to be a short-lived triumph. As of 2014, we are starting to age prematurely again in the UK, and this time, not because of the diseases we now traditionally consider to belong to old age, such as osteoarthritis or osteoporosis, but because of our failure to respect our metabolic capacity.

Industrialisation requires a ready workforce, regularly fed and in good health. The synergistic relationship between technological advancement, improved nutrition, physiological function, and ultimately, increased longevity is a well recognised trend throughout human history. From an evolutionary perspective, the resulting increases in population size are sustained by our ability to produce food more and more efficiently through employing increasingly specialised technologies. This has had a two-fold effect. Those individuals who suffer under-nutrition not only fail to thrive physiologically and have a reduced life expectancy but also have less energy to expend on labour for food production as well as social and technological advancement. Therefore, healthier, optimised bodies are a hallmark of a growing population and a thriving society. Our bodies have responded and continue to respond to the changing availability of calories and to the particular sources of the calories we consume in terms of physiological functioning and energy expenditure. The efficiency of the 'human engine', as Robert Fogel has coined the phrase, is estimated to have increased by about 53% between 1790 and 1980 in the UK, against the backdrop of a fourfold increase in the global population and exponential technological development over the past century.

It seems, however, that this bubble of an ever-improving quality and length of life might be about to burst. Industrialisation not only requires an expanding workforce but also thrives on increasing numbers of consumers. Today, many mass produced time-saving foods, drinks and other 'psychoactive' substances, such as tobacco and sugar, are big business for global markets and often bring us kudos and social gratification through perpetual bombardment by social media and the marketing of idealised lifestyles and identities. However, we also now know that these consumable substances, especially in abundance, are causing our bodies to fail, both genetically and physiologically. Obesity and type 2 diabetes are now significantly impacting our health as a population and foreshortening our lives, and this is particularly affecting economically deprived populations in the UK today, creating the effect of the 'metabolic ghetto'. As identified by Jonathan C. K. Wells, this is a cycle of the biological inability to tolerate metabolic overload, perpetuated over generations, through a reduced metabolic capacity resulting from maternal nutritional deficiencies *in utero* and foetal programming, simultaneously compounded by learned social behaviours related to urbanisation, such as sedentary lifestyles, consumption of fast food, diets high in sugar and social aspirations to the latest lifestyle choices. The resulting obesity, in particular visceral fat, exacerbates many life-shortening conditions that are common today.

Not only then did we transition from a dominance of infectious to non-communicable diseases during the 20th century but this period also represents a 'nutrition transition' in our epidemiological history, from a diet high in fibre and cereals to one high in sugars, trans-fats and animal-source food. Nutrition, and its functions of bodily growth, metabolism and repair, is now key to our longevity but its quality and substance is highly controlled by competitive international market producers. Sidney Mintz suggests that 'we are made into what we eat through forces of consumption and identity' and this is reflected by the fact that metabolic capacity, metabolic overload, consumer status, education and living standards are not equally distributed across the population. Today in the UK, those from better off areas not only live 10 years longer on average than those at a socio-economic disadvantage but also experience up to 20 years better health. London overall continues to see a rise in longevity, for example, compared to isolated rural and post-industrial areas.

As such, our health in the UK reflects wider economic strategies and in fact, biomedical statistics often reflect the true economic status of a population more accurately than the conventional economic tests, especially, according to Fogel, for investigating secular trends in inequality. Over time, our bodies have been manufactured into either instruments of labour or victims of profit. Londoners epitomise both extremes, in many cases still echoing the experience of health in the City 100 or 200 years ago. Human biology, social behaviours and history are inextricably intertwined via feedback loops in our cellular make-up and DNA that we even today we can barely separate but that we are destined to pass on to the next generation. These create unique experiences of health that feed into common geographic collectives. We, of course, as an innovative species, continue to adapt. Older populations and greater numbers of the elderly places a focus on the study of those illnesses integral to the burden of age, such as cancer, diabetes, cardiovascular disease, osteoarthritis, osteoporosis and dementia. Our study indicates that the skeletal manifestations of several of these conditions have increased over time in the old age population as a corollary of the industrialised aging process and increased numbers of 70+ year olds in modern populations. Genetic factors play an important role in ageing and age related diseases, contributing to the longevity of a person's life by the inheritance of genetic variations or their mutation over the lifetime that may protect or predispose an individual to the processes of disease. While increased funding and improvements to the state provision of pensions, social care and medical treatment in many countries is proven to improve overall population health, and in particular for those on lower incomes or with little family support, within the medical field, developments are now moving towards a regenerative medical approach, incorporating genetic research whereby investigation can be made at a molecular and cellular level to better understand our genetic propensity to accelerated aging and disease.

Research undertaken at the Centre for Ageing, Lancaster University, published in 2018, indicated that damage to DNA is a basis of ageing, causing an alteration to its structure and affecting normal processes in the body. Genetic studies based on animal models investigating ageing and senescent cells (unwanted cells that cease to divide), which may be triggered by damage to DNA and telomere shortening at the ends of chromosomes, have found that these cells increase in number within tissues of organs. Telomere shortening or attrition is still a rapidly expanding area of medical research, though to date has been widely accepted as being a part of, or maybe even contributing to, the ageing process, activated not only as we grow older but also accentuated by biological sex, ethnic affiliation and to a lesser extent by unhealthy diets, smoking, obesity, stress, metabolic syndrome, working conditions, inflammation and a lack of exercise. An increase in the rate of telomere shortening is associated with premature ageing. There is future potential in this area that could lead to the development of drugs to remove senescent cells in humans to enhance the functions in older individuals (senolytics) as well as to control the telomere shortening process through the modification of enzyme actions. However, of consideration is the fact that while starvation and malnutrition may have led to telomere shortening in the past, predisposing us to premature ageing, longer telomeres resulting from the improved food production that industrialisation brought not only extend life expectancy but are also a risk factor for certain cancers in modern populations. If the evolutionary hypothesis of the 'thrifty telomere' is correct, industrialisation has facilitated a transition from shorter to longer telomeres, which may be paternally inherited for the potential benefit of future generations but are not without consequences for human health in today's living environment.

This project's re-examination of the archaeological human remains from archives not only in London but across the country, emphasises both the importance of the retention of this unique source of evidence for how health has changed in response to environmental conditions as well as how the application of modern technologies can shine a light on new evidence lying previously undiscovered on dusty shelves. New techniques will continue to be explored and developed, especially with regards to DNA and biomolecular screening technologies to identify specific infections that we currently cannot detect, providing a wealth of objective evidence for health in the past that is currently unavailable. However, for the present time, the evidence we have amassed here using digital imaging demonstrates that the change in our living environments in Britain, from largely agrarian, rural lifestyles to those based on heavy industry and technology, has left a deeply embedded imprint on many aspects of our health in London and the wider UK today. The biological changes we observe in archaeological human remains are a testament to how we are responsible for manufacturing our living environments and our bodies as a result, and by comparing this evidence from the past, we will be able to continue to trace the re-manufacturing of our bodies in the future. What will health have been like in post-industrial London? Watch this space!

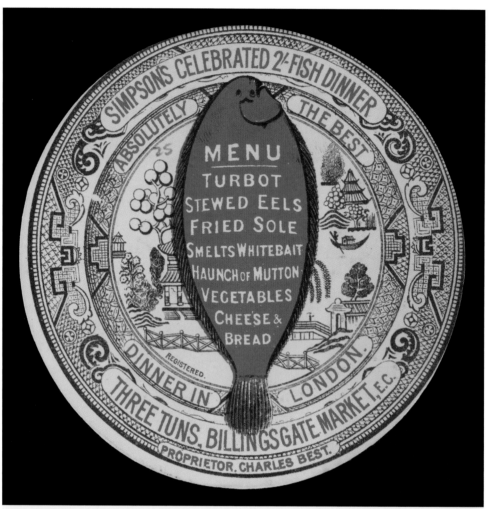

Figure 198 Advertisement for Simpsons Fish Dinner at the Three Tuns, Billingsgate Market, London
(Credit: Wellcome Collection, cc-by/4.0)

Further information and details relating to the research project can be found at
http://www.museumoflondon.org.uk/manufacturedbodies

Glossary of terms

Age-standardised rate of mortality – Age-standardised mortality rate is a weighted average of the age-specific mortality rates per 100,000 persons. Age standardisation is a technique used to allow populations from different parts of a country to be compared fairly. For example, if 60% of the national population is 50+ years old, all the mortality rates for each individual geographic area will be adjusted so that this age group represents 60% of the population in each geographic area. Once the statistics are corrected, there can be no biases in mortality rates caused by differences in the age compositions of each population

Body Mass Index –An approximate measure of whether someone is over or underweight; calculated by dividing their weight in kilograms by the square of their height in metres

CT – Computerised tomography. More detailed information can be provided by CT scans than radiographs, as the scans combine a series of images taken from different angles and use computer processing to create cross-sectional images (slices) of the bones that can be further processed to create 3D images. In comparison, radiographs are only 2D images.

Digital radiography – Digital x-rays

Epigenetic – Non-genetic influences on the gene expression by biological mechanisms that affect how genes are read by cells and which genes are switched on and off

Low status and High status – The social status of some sites in Industrial London is identifiable from historic records and archaeological information. Crypt burial, for example, is associated with wealthier of society equating to high status, in addition to any expensive accompanying grave furniture. More basic burial in poorer locations in London is an indication that an individual's social status is likely to be low. In this study, Chelsea, Mare Street in Hackney and St Bride's Crypt are considered high status from their location and burial types. Conversely, burials from Bow, Bethnal Green and St Bride's lower burial ground are considered as low status

Mortality rate – The percentage of deaths in a particular population in relation to specific causes

N – Within tables presenting data, N is the total sample number

n – Within tables presenting data, n is the number of cases affected

Percentage (%) Fraction – Percentage of the fraction of all-cause mortality attributable to a particular cause having contributed to deaths, statistically modelled according to the relative presence of the risk factor in each population

Prevalence – Refers to the number of cases of a disease that are present in a particular population over a given period of time in the past

Resection – Cutting out tissue or part of an organ

Selected further reading

General

Ackroyd, P. (2011). *London Under*. London: Vintage Books.

Fogel, R. W. (2004). *The Escape from Hunger and Premature Death, 1700–2100: Europe, America, and the Third World*. Cambridge: Cambridge University Press.

Lewis, J. (1988). *London the Autobiography*. London: Constable and Robinson.

Mayhew, H. (1851). *London Labour and the London Poor*. Vols 1–3. New York: Harper & Brothers.

Porter, R. (2000). *London: A Social History*. London: Penguin Books.

Thane, P. (2000). *Old Age in English History: past experiences, present issues*. Oxford: Oxford University Press.

Werner, A. (ed.) (1998). *London Bodies: changing shape of londoners from prehistoric times to the present day*. London: Museum of London.

Wells, J. C. K. (2016). *The Metabolic Ghetto: an evolutionary perspective on nutrition, power relations and chronic disease*. Cambridge: Cambridge University Press

Chapter 1: Occupational hazards and sporting catastrophes

Crossley, D. W. (ed.) (1981). *Medieval Industry*. London: Council for British Archaeology Research Report 40.

Driver and Vehicle Standards Agency. (2018). *History of Road Safety, The Highway Code and the Driving Test*. [On Line] Available at https://www.gov.uk/government/publications/history-of-road-safety-and-the-driving-test/history-of-road-safety-the-highway-code-and-the-driving-test

Guttman, A. (1991). *Women's Sports: a history*. Columbia OH: Columbia University Press.

Haley, B. (1978). *The Healthy Body and Victorian Culture*. Cambridge MA and London: Harvard University Press.

Health and Safety Executive. (2018). *Workplace Fatal Injuries in Great Britain 2018*. [On Line] Available from www.hse.gov.uk/statistics

Health and Safety Executive. (2018). *The History of HSE*. [On Line] Available at http://www.hse.gov.uk/aboutus/timeline/index.htm

Leigh. S. (1830). *Leigh's New Picture of London*. London: Leigh.

Mckaye, B. (2009). *Boxing: a manly history of the sweet science of bruising*. [On Line] Available at https://www.artofmanliness.com/articles/boxing-a-manly-history-of-the-sweet-science-of-bruising/

Pedroche, B. (2013). *Working the London Underground from 1863 to 2013*. Stroud: History Press.

Simkin, J. (2015). *History of Football*. [On Line] Available at https://spartacus-educational.com/Fhistory.htm

Chapter 2: The air we breathe

Brignall, M. (2018). Burning issue: are wood-burning stoves going to get the chop? *The Guardian* (26 May) Available at https://www.theguardian.com/money/2018/may/26/wood-burner-open-fire-pollution-cleaning-up-air-quality

Brimblecombe, P. (1976). Attitudes and responses towards air pollution in medieval England. *Journal of the Air Pollution Control Association.* 26(10), 941-945. [On Line] Available at: https://doi.org/10.1080/00022470.1976.10470341

Chen, W., Liu, Y., Huang, X. and Rong, Y. (2012). Respiratory diseases among dust exposed workers. In Ghanei, M. (ed.) *Respiratory Diseases.* IntechOpen DOI: 10.5772/32357. [On Line] Available at https://www.intechopen.com/books/respiratory-diseases/respiratory-diseases-among-dust-exposed-workers

Evans, S. (2015). *UK Coal Use to Fall to Lowest Level Since Industrial Revolution. Carbon Brief Clear on Climate.* [On Line] Available at https://www.carbonbrief.org/uk-coal-use-to-fall-to-lowest-level-since-industrial-revolution

Green, M. (2017). When London was the Smoking Capital of the World. *The Telegraph* (7th March). [On Line] Available at https://www.telegraph.co.uk/travel/destinations/europe/united-kingdom/england/london/articles/The-surprising-history-of-Londons-lost-tobacco-houses/

Health and Safety Executive. (2018). *Pneumoconiosis* [On Line]. Available at http://www.hse.gov.uk/lung-disease/pneumoconiosis.htm

Hilton, M. (2000). *Smoking in British Popular Culture.* New York: Manchester University Press.

Intriguing History. *Gas Lights and the Lamplighters of London, the Glow of Victorian London.* [On Line] Available at http://www.intriguing-history.com/gas-lights-lamplighters/

Peto, R., Darby, S., Deo, H., Silcocks, P, Whitley, E. and Doll, R. (2000). Smoking, smoking cessation and lung cancer in the UK since 1950: combination of national statistics with two case-control studies. *British Medical Journal.* 321, 323–9.

Philips, D., Osmond, C., Southall, H., Aucott, P., Jones, A. and Holgate, S. (2018). Evaluating the long-term consequences of air pollution in early life: geographical correlations between coal consumption in 1951/1952 and current mortality in England and Wales. *British Medical Journal Open.* 8:e018231. [On Line] Available at https://bmjopen.bmj.com/content/8/4/e018231

Chapter 3: Cancer

Cancer Research UK. [On Line] https://www.cancerresearchuk.org/ [Accessed 18 Jun 2018]

Hunt: K., Roberts, C. and Kirkpatrick, C. (2018). Taking stock: a systematic review of archaeological evidence of cancers in human and early hominin remains. *International Journal of Paleopathology* 21, 12–26.

Kyle, R. 2000. Multiple myeloma: an odyssey of discovery. *British Journal of Haematology* 111, 1035–44.

Moscucci, O. (2005). Gender and cancer in Britain, 1860–1910. *American Journal of Public Health* 95, 1312–21.

NHS England. (2014). *Five Year Cancer Commissioning Strategy for London.* [On Line] Available at https://www.england.nhs.uk/london/wp-content/uploads/sites/8/2014/04/london-5yr-cancer-comm-strategy.pdf

Reddington, J., Mendez, G., Ching, A., Kubicky, C., Klimo, P. and Ragel, B. (2016). Imaging characteristic analysis of metastatic spine lesions from breast, prostate, lung and renal cell carcinomas for surgical planning: osteolytic v osteoblastic. *Surgical Neurology International*. 7, S361–5. [On Line] Available at https://www.ncbi.nlm.nih.gov/pmc/articles/PMC4879848/

Riaz, S., Horton, M., Kang, J., Mak, V., Lüchtenborg, M. and Møller, H. (2011). Lung cancer incidence and survival in England: an analysis by socioeconomic deprivation and urbanization. *Journal of Thoracic Oncology* 6, 2005–10.

University of Pittsburgh Schools of Health Sciences. (2017) Telomere Length Predicts Cancer Risk. *Science Daily*, 3 April. [On Line] Available at https://www.sciencedaily.com/releases/2017/04/170403083123.htm

Weiss, L. (2000). Concepts of metastasis. *Cancer and Metastasis Reviews* 19, 219–34.

Chapter 4: Getting fat: a growing crisis

Carlin, M. and Rosenthal, J. (1998). *Food and Eating in Medieval Europe.* London: Hambledon.

Clayton, P. and Rowbotham, J. (2009). How the mid-Victorians worked, ate and died. *International Journal of Environmental Research and Public Health* 6, 1235–53. [On Line] Available at https://www.ncbi.nlm.nih.gov/pmc/articles/PMC2672390/

Deng, T, Lyon, C.J, Bergin, S, Caligiuri, M.A, and Hsueh W. A. 2016. Obesity, inflammation, and cancer. *Annual Review of Pathology* 11 (May), 421–49.

Gilman, S. (2010). *Obesity: the biography.* Oxford: Oxford University Press.

Mintz, S. (1986). *Sweetness and Power.* New York: Penguin Books.

Pasquali, R. (2005). Obesity and androgens: facts and perspectives. *American Society for Reproductive Medicine* 85 (5), 1319–40.

Public Health England. (2014). *Adult Obesity and Type 2 Diabetes.* Available at https://assets.publishing.service.gov.uk/government/uploads/system/uploads/attachment_data/file/338934/Adult_obesity_and_type_2_diabetes_.pdf [Accessed 5 Jul.2018]

Symons, M. (2004). *A History of Cooks and Cooking.* Urbana and Chicago IL: University of Illinois Press.

Tattersall, R. (2009). *Diabetes: the biography.* Oxford: Oxford University Press.

Western, A. and Bekvalac, J. (2017). Hyperostosis Frontalis Interna in female historic skeletal populations: age, sex hormones and the impact of industrialization. *American Journal of Physical Anthropology.* 162 (3), 501–15. [On Line] Available at https://onlinelibrary.wiley.com/doi/abs/10.1002/ajpa.23133

Chapter 5: Growing old: us in winter clothes

Arthritis Research UK [On Line] Available at https://www.arthritisresearchuk.org/ [Accessed 3 Dec. 2018]

Barnett, E. and Nordin, B.E.(1960). The radiological diagnosis of osteoporosis: a new approach. *Clinical Radiology* 11 (July), 166–74.

Broderick, D. (1999). *The Last Mortal Generation.* Sydney: New Holland.

Chadwick, E. (1842). Report on the sanitary conditions of the labouring population of Great Britain, 1842. London: House of Commons Sessional Paper

Chase, K. (2009). *Victorians and Old Age.* Oxford: Oxford University Press.

Eisenberg, D, T. (2011). An evolutionary review of human telomere biology: the thrifty telomere hypothesis and notes on potential adaptive paternal effects. *American Journal of Human Biology.* 23 (2), 149–67.

Griffin, E. (2018). Diets, hunger and living standards during the British Industrial Revolution. *Past and Present* 239 (1), 71–111.

Haara, M, Heliövaar, M, Impivaara, O, Arokoski, J. P, Manninen, P, Knekt, P, Kärkkäinen, A, Reunanen, A, Aromaa, A and Kröger, H. (2006). Low metacarpal index predicts hip fracture: a prospective population study of 3,561 subjects with 15 years of follow-up. *Acta Orthopaedica* 77 (1), 9–14

Office for National Statistics 2014–2016. Available at https://www.ons.gov.uk/releases/healthstate lifeexpectanciesuk2014to2016

Public Health England. 2011–12. *Knee and Hip osteoarthritis.* [On Line] Available at http://www. arthritisresearchuk.org/arthritis-information/data-and-statistics.aspx

Roberts, C.A. and Cox, M. (2003). *Health and Disease in Britain from Prehistory to the Present Day.* Stroud: Sutton.

Shahar, S. (2004). *Growing Old in the Middle Ages.* London: Routledge.

Tanner, D.A, Kloseck, M, Crilly, R.G, Chesworth, B, Gilliland, J. (2010). Hip fracture types in men and women change differently with age. *BMC Geriatrics*, 10, 12 [On Line] Available at https://doi.org/10.1186/1471-2318-10-12

The Royal Osteoporosis Society. [On Line] Available at https://theros.org.uk/ [Accessed 15 Feb. 2019]

United Nations Population Fund [On Line] Available at https://www.unfpa.org/ [Accessed 1 Nov. 2018]

Walker, D. (2012). London's volcanic winter: Spitalfields cemetery and the famine of 1258. *Current Archaeology* 370, 12–19.

Site monographs and unpublished site reports

Alexander, M., Austick, J., Buglass, J., Caffell, A., Fackrell, M., Fackrell, K., French, M., Goodall, C., Gowland, R., Hart, M., Holst, M., Heyworth, B., Lister, A., Lister, M., Monaghan, C., Monaghan, M., Neal, S., Power, D. (2017). *The Fewston Assemblage: churchyard secrets revealed.* Washburn: Washburn Heritage Centre.

Boucher, A., Craddock-Bennet, L. and Daly, T. (2015). *Death in the Close: a medieval mystery.* Edinburgh: Headland Archaeology (UK) Ltd.

Connell, B., Gray Jones, A., Redfern, R., and Walker, D. (2012). *A Bioarchaeological Study of Medieval burials on the site of St Mary Spital: excavations at Spitalfields Market, London E1, 1991-2007.* London: Museum of London Archaeology Monograph 60.

Grainger, I and Phillpotts, C. (2011). *The Cistercian Abbey of St Mary Graces, East Smithfield, London.* London: Museum of London Archaeology 44.

Henderson, M., Miles, A, Walker, D. with Connell, B, and Wroe-Brown, R. (2013). *'He being dead yet speaketh': excavations at three post-medieval burial grounds in Tower Hamlets, east London, 2004-10.* London: Museum of London Archaeology 64.

Johnson, L. (undated). *History of Scaife Farm.* [On Line] Available at https://scaifehallfarm.co.uk/historyofscaifehallfarm.pdf

Mays, S., Harding, C. and Heighway, C. (2007). *Wharram, A Study of Settlement on the Yorkshire Wolds XI: the churchyard.* York: York University Archaeological Publication 13.

Miles, A. and Carty, N. (forthcoming). *Mare Street Baptist Church Burial Ground: excavations at 143 Mare Street, London E8, 2014.* London: Museum of London Archaeology.

Oxford Archaeology North, (forthcoming) *The Swinton Unitarian Free Chapel Cemetery, Swinton, Greater Manchester.*

Proctor, J., Gaimster, M. and Langthorne, J. (2016). *A Quaker Burial Ground in North Shields: Excavations at Coach Lane, Tyne and Wear.* Where published: Pre-Construct Archaeology Monograph 20.

Schofield, J., Blackmore, L. and Pearce, J. with Dyson, T. (2019). *London's Waterfront 1100–1666: excavations in Thames Street, London, 1974-84.* Oxford: Archaeopress.

Telford, A. and Knox, E. (forthcoming). *'Under the Roof and the Shadow of a Noble Church': archaeological investigation at St George's, Brentford, 2014–2017.* London: Museum of London Archaeology.

Waldron, T. (2007). *St Peter's, Barton-upon-Humber, Lincolnshire: a parish church and its community. Volume 2: the human remains.* Oxford: Oxbow Books.

Wessex Archaeology (2017) *New Covent Garden Market Entrance Site (Nine Elms Gardens), Nine Elms Lane, London Borough of Wandsworth: post-excavation assessment and updated project design for analysis and publication.* Salisbury: unpublished client report 107903.04.

Western, A. G. (2016). *Osteological Analysis of the Human Remains from the South Side of Holy Trinity Church, Old Town, Stratford-upon-Avon, Warwickshire.* Unpublished Ossafreelance Report OA1063. [On Line] Available at https://ossafreelance.co.uk/wp/commercial-reports/

Western, A. G. (2014). *Osteological Analysis of Human Remains from the Old Church of St. Peter and St. Paul, Upton-on-Severn, Worcestershire.* Unpublished Ossafreelance Report. OA1044. [On Line] Available at https://ossafreelance.co.uk/wp/commercial-reports/

Index